Echocardiogram Profiles after Acute Myocardial Infarction

ZEEV VLODAVER

ECHOCARDIOGRAM PROFILES AFTER ACUTE MYOCARDIAL INFARCTION

by
ZEEV VLODAVER, M.D.
Director, Section Noninvasive Cardiology
and Cardiac Rehabilitation

Unity Medical Center
Fridley, Minnesota

and the collaboration of

BRADLEY M. NELSON, A.S.
Chief Echo Technician
Unity Medical Center

ALLAN BOYUM, M.D.,
SIM GESUNDHEIT, M.D.,
STEVEN LONG, M.D.,
ROBERT PETERSON, M.D.,
EDWARD A. SPENNY, M.D., and
R. DOUGLAS THORSEN, M.D.
Department of Medicine
Unity Medical Center

KATHY HANSEN, O.T.R.,
TOM LITECKY, B.A.,
YVONNE LYRENMANN, O.T.R.,
BEVERLY SCHMIT, R.N., and
CAROL WIEGREFE, R.D.,
Cardiac rehabilitation Team
Unity Medical Center

PAUL GANNON, M.D.
EVAN F. LINDBERG, M.D.
Thoracic and Cardiovascular Surgeons
Minneapolis, Minnesota

Ishiyaku EuroAmerica, Inc./Medical Series
Carlo P. Caciolo, M.D., Advisor
Allen D. Soffer, M.D., Advisor
Antonio H.M. Salvador, M.D., Advisor (Pathology)

Ishiyaku EuroAmerica, Inc.
11559 Rock Island Court, St. Louis, Missouri 63043

Library of Congress Catalogue Card Number 84-27840

Vlodaver, Zeev
    Echocardiogram Profiles after Acute Myocardial Infarction

ISBN 0-912791-07-1

Printed in the United States of America

Ishiyaku EuroAmerica, Inc.
St. Louis • Tokyo

Composition and design: Graphic World, Inc., St. Louis, Missouri
Printed by Malloy Lithographing, Inc., Ann Arbor, Michigan

PREFACE

The goal of this book is to provide a comprehensive overview of echocardiography and its usefulness in the evaluation of the patient with acute myocardial infarction. The book is designed for the person who deals in day-to-day practice with this common clinical problem in the fields of cardiology, internal medicine, cardiac rehabilitation and nursing, as well as the student and practitioners who are trying to increase their knowledge of echocardiography.

An introductory chapter presents normal LV echocardiogram patterns and technical approaches with M-Mode and two-dimensional echocardiography. Specific chapters address the subjects of echocardiographic patterns in acute myocardial infarction and the evaluation of its complications. A major section deals with a patient's clinical progress, and with LV echocardiogram profiles throughout the various stages of a cardiac rehabilitation program.

Another important chapter discusses surgical "revascularization" with indications and post-operative states, and the surgical treatment of myocardial infarction and its sequelae.

The seeds for coronary heart disease may be present in early life, with changes and possible differences in various ethnic groups. These alterations of the norm in the coronary arteries may predispose to coronary atherosclerosis. Therefore, we could not conclude this work without emphasizing the importance of recognizing these changes in young people.

ACKNOWLEDGEMENTS

While it is not possible to name all who in one way or another have contributed to this book, the author wishes to express appreciation to all who have had an influence upon the production of the final work.

At Unity Medical Center, a community hospital in Fridley, Minnesota, an atmosphere was established wherein the studies necessary for this work could be done in an unhampered manner.

For this, we are grateful to Mr. John F. Haines, Executive Vice President, and Mr. John R. Murphy, Vice President, of Unity Medical Center, a division of the Health Central System and to its administration. Thanks are expressed to internists Drs. Robert Engebretson, Jan D. Johnson, John W. Lawrow, Alexander Levitan, Harold Londer, and John Kleinman, who referred patients for Cardiac Rehabilitation and Echocardiography after thorough clinical evaluation.

We are appreciative of the efforts and cooperation of Dr. James Daniel, Cardiologist, and Jeanne Olson, Chief Echocardiogram Technician from Abbott-Northwestern Hospital, who provided us with some of the echocardiograms used in this book.

We recognize with appreciation and are deeply indebted to Betty Koerner for her work in proofreading the manuscript and providing editorial criticism. Thanks also go to Corinne Copeland for the typing of this manuscript and charts.

TABLE OF CONTENTS

Table of Contents

LIST OF ABBREVIATIONS

LV	Left Ventricle
RV	Right Ventricle
LA	Left Atrium
RA	Right Atrium
Ao	Aorta
IVS	Interventricular Septum
PW	Posterior Wall
Th	Thrombus
CRP	Cardiac Rehabilitation Program
EF	Ejection Fraction
Mean VCF	Mean Velocity of Circumferential Fiber Shortening
Δ % thick	Percentage of Thickening
↓	Reduced
↑	Increased
LVD	LV Internal Dimension in Diastole
Aneu	Aneurysm
ECG	Electrocardiogram
AV	Aortic Valve
PV	Pulmonic Valve
MV	Mitral Valve
TV	Tricuspid Valve
KHz	Kilohertz
MHz	Megahertz
PMI	Point of Maximal Impulse
LC	Left Coronary Artery
RC	Right Coronary Artery
LAD	Left Anterior Descending Coronary Artery

B. M-Mode Echocardiography

Important left ventricular regions not visualized by M-mode techniques:

1. True posterior or inferior wall.

2. Lateral or free wall segments.

3. Apical segments.

B. M-Mode Echocardiography

Normal M-mode echocardiogram:

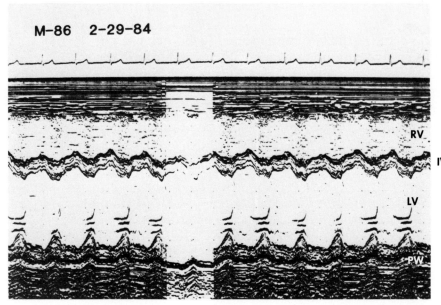

Fig. 1. A, M-mode LV echocardiogram demonstrating normal motion of the IVS and posterior wall of the LV. The dimensions of the RV and LV in diastole and systole are normal.

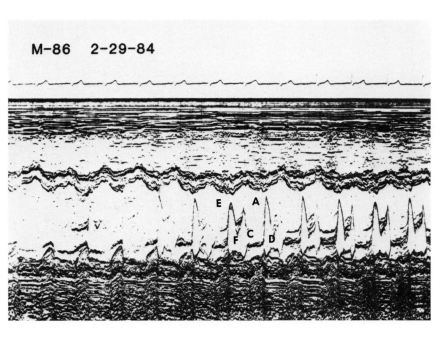

Fig. 1. B, M-mode scan with normal mitral valve. Point **E** represents maximal opening of the mitral valve in early diastole. Slope **E** to **F** indicates closing velocity of the mitral valve, and the **A** wave is the atrial contribution to ventricular filling. The **C-D** interval represents left ventricular systole.

C. Two-Dimensional Echocardiography

Two-dimensional echocardiography uses ultrasound to create a cross-section imaging plane that enables us to take tomographic sections of the heart at many different levels from a number of different locations on the chest.

Using a number of different imaging planes, the two-dimensional technique allows the study of anatomic spacial relationships of the left ventricle. The symmetry or asymmetry of left ventricular contraction can be documented along with the identification of regional wall motion abnormalities.

The cross-section plane of the two-dimensional technique enables us to visualize regions of myocardium previously undetectable with the M-mode technique and allows the detection and diagnosis of ventricular aneurysms with greater ease and certainty.

There are six major views important in the study of the coronary artery disease patient and the patient with an acute myocardial infarction.

C. Two-Dimensional Echocardiography

1. *Parasternal Long Axis View*

The patient is usually examined in the partial left lateral decubitus position. The transducer is placed on the left sternal border, third-to-fourth intercostal space, with the imaging plane approximately parallel to a line joining the right shoulder and the left flank. The image produced is a cross-section of the left ventricle through its long axis. The orientation of this image is such that the aorta is on the right and the left ventricle and axis are toward the left. Anteriorly, we find the chest wall and right ventricle.

The parasternal long axis view nicely visualizes the anterior portion of the interventricular septum, left ventricular posterior wall, mitral valve, aortic valve, aortic root and left atrium. A small portion of the right ventricle and the right ventricular anterior wall are also visualized.

C. Two-Dimensional Echocardiography

1. *Parasternal Long Axis View*

Usually only ⅔ to ¾ of the left ventricle is visualized in this view. Due to the parasternal location of the transducer, the apical portion of the left ventricle is usually difficult to image from this position.

It should be noted that the M-mode echocardiogram recordings are taken while tilting the single crystal transducer along this same imaging plane.

C. Two-Dimensional Echocardiography

1. *Parasternal Long Axis View*

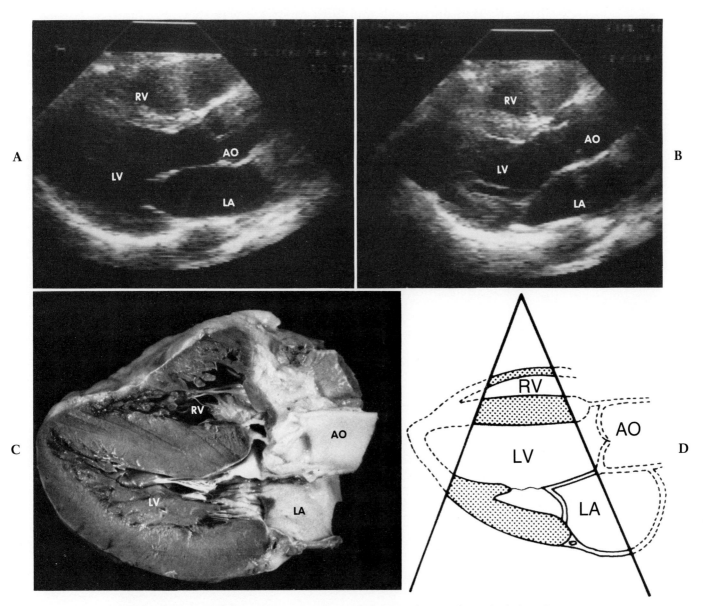

Fig. 2. Parasternal long axis recording of the LV during diastole (**A**) and systole (**B**). The dimensions of the chambers LV, RV and LA are normal. In real time, motion and systolic thickening also are normal. The accompanying specimen (**C**) and diagram (**D**) illustrate the long axis view. Fig. 2D used with permission of the American Heart Association Inc. from Walter L. Henry, Anthony DeMaria, Raimond Gramiak, Donald L. King, Joseph A. Kisslo, Richard L. Popp, David J. Sahn, Nelson B. Schiller, Abdul Tajik, Lewis E. Teichholz and Arthur E. Weyman. Circ. 62:212, 1980.

C. Two-Dimensional Echocardiography

2. *Parasternal Short Axis View*

From the long axis position, the imaging plane is rotated 90° clock-wise producing a cross-section of the left ventricle along its short axis. By tilting the transducer back and forth in such a way that the plane of the tilting motion is perpendicular to the imaging plane, we can scan the left ventricle from the base toward the apex.

The parasternal short axis view is divided into three cross-sectional levels of the left ventricle.

1) Basilar Region: At approximately the level of the mitral valve, the entire septum, and anterior, posterior, inferior and lateral walls of the left ventricle can be examined for symmetry or asymmetry of motion and contraction. The right ventricular walls can also be visualized from this level.

2) Mid Ventricular Region: This is a short axis plane of the left ventricle at the level of the papillary muscles.

3) Apical Region: This is the short axis plane at the level just below the papillary muscles of the left ventricle.

C. Two-Dimensional Echocardiography

2. *Parasternal Short Axis View*

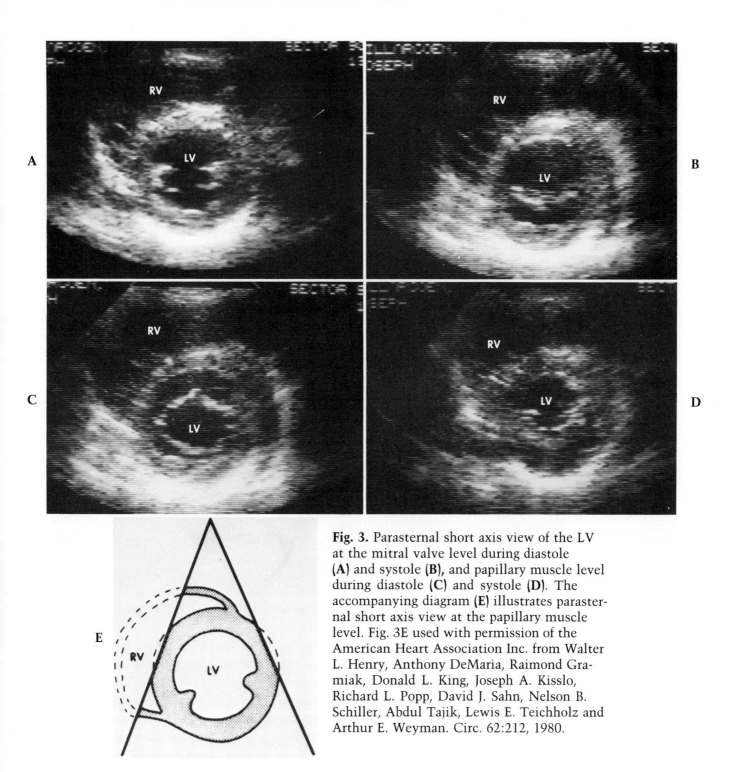

Fig. 3. Parasternal short axis view of the LV at the mitral valve level during diastole (**A**) and systole (**B**), and papillary muscle level during diastole (**C**) and systole (**D**). The accompanying diagram (**E**) illustrates parasternal short axis view at the papillary muscle level. Fig. 3E used with permission of the American Heart Association Inc. from Walter L. Henry, Anthony DeMaria, Raimond Gramiak, Donald L. King, Joseph A. Kisslo, Richard L. Popp, David J. Sahn, Nelson B. Schiller, Abdul Tajik, Lewis E. Teichholz and Arthur E. Weyman. Circ. 62:212, 1980.

C. Two-Dimensional Echocardiography

2. *Parasternal Short Axis View*

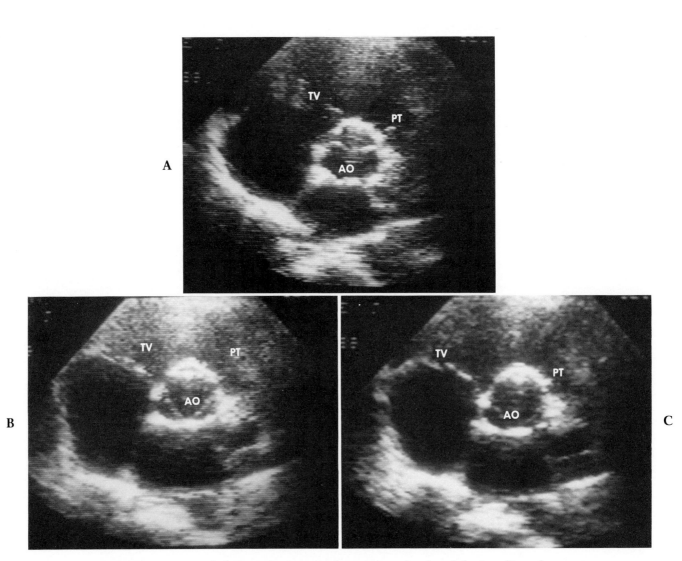

Fig. 4. Parasternal short axis view at the aortic valve level during diastole (**A**), early systole (**B**) and late systole (**C**).

C. Two-Dimensional Echocardiography

3. *Apical Four-Chamber View*

The patient's position is similar to that needed for the parasternal views. The transducer is placed over the cardiac apex, more specifically over the PMI. The ultrasound beam is directed medially and superiorly toward the patient's right scapula. Orientation is such that all four chambers of the heart are visualized along with both A-V valves. The left ventricle and left atrium are usually displayed on the right side of the screen and the cardiac apex at the top of the screen.

This view enables us to study the anterolateral left ventricular free wall as well as the inferior portion of the interventricular septum. The left ventricular apex is nicely visualized from this position. It is extremely important that the left ventricular apex be studied thoroughly, especially in those patients with anteroseptal infarctions. Apical aneurysms and thrombi can often be detected in this view.

A variation of the apical four-chamber can be obtained by angling the imaging plane inferiorly from the standard four-chamber view. This approach enables us to study the symmetry or asymmetry of the inferior and posterior walls quite near the base. This area can be difficult to study at times with other standard views. The apical four-chamber view with inferior angulation can be very helpful in the study of basalar infarctions.

C. Two-Dimensional Echocardiography

4. *Apical Two-Chamber View*

From the standard apical four-chamber position, the imaging plane is rotated approximately 70 degrees counter-clockwise. The mitral valve, left atrium and the anterior free wall, apex and inferior wall of the left ventricle are visualized. Orientation is such that the anterior wall is displayed on the right, inferior wall on the left.

C. Two-Dimensional Echocardiography

5. *Apical Long Axis View*

From the standard apical four-chamber position, the imaging plane is rotated approximately 90 degrees counter-clockwise. This view allows the study of anterior ventricular septum, apex and posterior wall of the left ventricular. Mitral valve, left atrium and aortic valve are also visualized. The orientation of this view displays the anterior septum on the right and the left ventricular posterior wall on the left.

C. Two-Dimensional Echocardiography

5. *Apical Long Axis View*

A

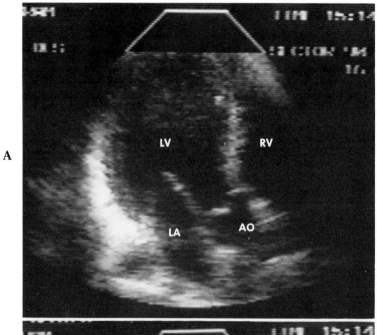

B

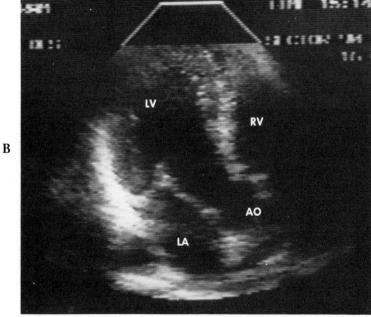

Fig. 7. Apical long axis view of the LV during diastole (**A**) and systole (**B**). The accompanying diagram (**C**), illustrates the apical long axis view in systole. Fig. 7C used with permission of the American Heart Association Inc. from Walter L. Henry, Anthony DeMaria, Raimond Gramiak, Donald L. King, Joseph A. Kisslo, Richard L. Popp, David J. Sahn, Nelson B. Schiller, Abdul Tajik, Lewis E. Teichholz and Arthur E. Weyman. Circ. 62:212, 1980.

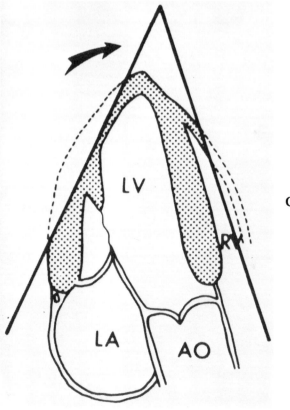

C

C. Two-Dimensional Echocardiography

6. *Subcostal View:*

The subcostal or subxiphoid approach may be the only cardiac image obtainable when there is poor ultrasound penetration in the parasternal and apical views. Patients with chronic obstructive lung disease usually have hyperinflated lungs which can obliterate parasternal and apical windows.

The patient is supine. The transducer position is just caudal to the xiphoid process and the imaging plane is directed superiorly and toward the patient's left and is then rotated until it is parallel to the long axis of the left ventricle. The right ventrical, right atrium and tricuspid valve are visualized anteriorly while posteriorly we have the left ventricle, left atrium and mitral valve. This view can be compared to the apical four-chamber view.

Specific myocardial regions visualized are those of the lateral and inferoseptal walls of the left ventricle and the left ventricular apex. The inferior right ventricular free wall can be visualized subcostally which can be an important view in cases of anteroseptal myocardial infarctions that could extend into the right ventricle.

The subcostal view is also used to detect some types of ventricular aneurysms and to study the right ventricular free wall in cases of cardiac tamponade.

C. Two-Dimensional Echocardiography

6. *Subcostal View:*

Relative cardiac chamber dimensions are also noted from this view.

Since both ventricles are nicely visualized from the subcostal approach, along with the interventricular septum, this is usually an excellent view for documenting a contrast echocardiogram. One possibility for a contrast echocardiogram would be to document an acquired ventricular septal defect due to a ruptured interventricular septum.

C. Two-Dimensional Echocardiography

6. *Subcostal View*

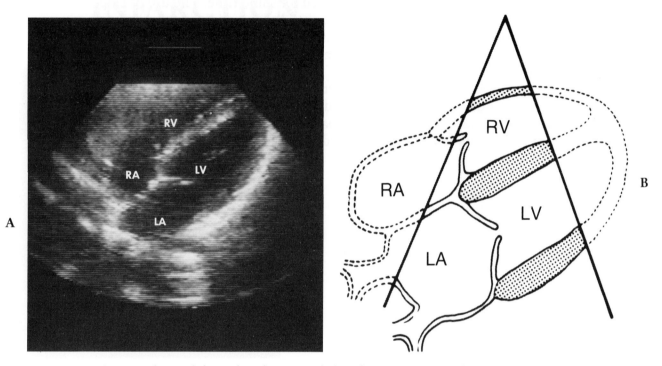

Fig. 8. Subcostal four-chamber view (**A**) and accompanying diagram (**B**) during systole. Fig. 8B used with permission of the American Heart Association Inc. from Walter L. Henry, Anthony DeMaria, Raimond Gramiak, Donald L. King, Joseph A. Kisslo, Richard L. Popp, David J. Sahn, Nelson B. Schiller, Abdul Tajik, Lewis E. Teichholz and Arthur E. Weyman. Circ. 62:212, 1980.

A. Definition

Myocardial infarction is necrosis of the cardiac muscle, as a complication of acute ischemia. This acute ischemic event may be precipitated by thrombosis occluding a coronary artery. Usually, severe atherosclerotic lesions are found in multiple foci.

The clinical diagnosis of myocardial infarction is based on severe and prolonged chest pain, with perspiration, dyspnea and anxiety. Electrocardiographic abnormalities are of ST-T segment changes, as well as QRS abnormalities (Q waves); and blood tests will detect a rise in the serum enzymes released by the injured myocardium (isoenzymes of creatinine phosphokinase (CPK-MB 130 enzyme) and of lactic acid dehydrogenase (LDH), important for the documentation of the diagnosis.

Death from ventricular arrhythmias is common in the first few hours if the patient is unattended.

Classically, there is mild fever and leukocytosis for 3 to 4 days, and pericardial friction rub can be heard in many of the patients with extensive infarction.

Post infarction pericarditis is generally benign, but temperature elevation, with severe distress and cardiac tamponade, can occur.

In some instances of acute myocardial infarction, the symptoms are mild, or atypical, and unrecognized by the patient (silent or atypical infarction).

Patients admitted to coronary care units with a diagnosis of acute myocardial infarction have regional wall motion abnormalities, associated with the area of myocardial damage, that can be detected with M-mode and two-dimensional echocardiography.

These wall motion abnormalities are commonly described as decreased amplitude of motion during systole, reduced systolic thickening and systolic thinning of the infarcted area.

Exaggerated wall motion is seen in the noninfarcted areas, particularly in the opposite wall, representing a compensatory hyperactivity.

A. Definition

A study of a group of patients with final diagnosis of acute infarction showed:

1. ECG (Minnesota Code Criteria for Acute MI) was diagnostic in 48% within 24 hours and in 65% of the patients after 24 hours of admission.

2. Enzymes CPK-MB isoenzymes were elevated: positive in 61%, trace in 13% in the first 24 hours. After 24 hours, they became positive in an additional 35% of the patients.

3. Two-dimensional echocardiogram (segmental LV motion and contraction abnormalities) was diagnostic in 86% of the patients in the first 24 hours.

Two-dimensional echocardiogram has higher sensitivity to other tests within 24 hours of admission and the highest specificity for recognition of location and extension of infarcted area.

The CPK-MB isoenzyme has the highest sensitivity and specificity for diagnosis of injury within 48 hours of admission but poor correlation with extension of injury.

ECG as a single test was diagnostic in only two-thirds of the patients. A normal or non-diagnostic ECG does not exclude acute infarction.

B. Anatomic Locations of Infarction

Myocardial infarction may involve either the full thickness of the LV, called transmural, or only the subendocardial portion of the wall, called subendocardial infarction.

If the whole heart is sectioned into five horizontal slices of approximately equal thickness, from apex to base (slice 1 is apical; slice 5 is basal), the infarctions can be classified according to their location as follows: anteroseptal, anterobasal, anterolateral, lateral, inferior, inferobasal, inferolateral, inferolateral basal, septal, apical and circumferential (See Figure 9.)

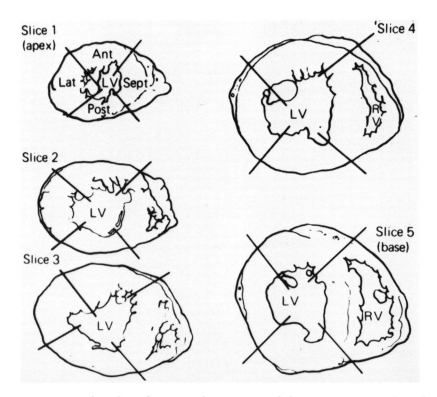

Fig. 9. Diagrams for identification of segments of the LV. Fig. 9 used with permission of Springer-Verlag New York Inc. from Coronary Heart Disease, Clinical, Angiographic and Pathologic Profile, 1976 by Vlodaver Z., Amplatz K., Burchell H. B. and Edwards J. E.

B. Anatomic Locations of Infarction

1. Anteroseptal Infarction
Located in the anterior wall, including the septum, slices 1 to 3.

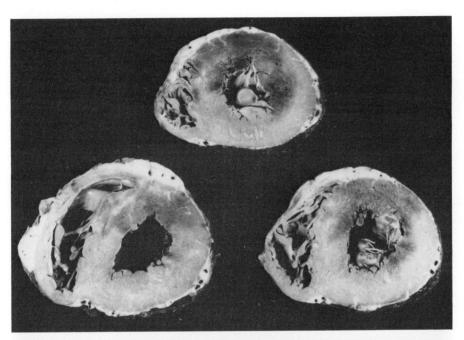

Fig. 10. Cross-section of the ventricular portion of the heart, showing discoloration of the anteroseptal segment of the LV 10 hours after acute myocardial infarction. Fig. 10 used with permission of Springer-Verlag New York Inc. from Coronary Heart Disease, Clinical, Angiographic and Pathologic Profile, 1976 by Vlodaver Z., Amplatz K., Burchell H. B. and Edwards J. E.

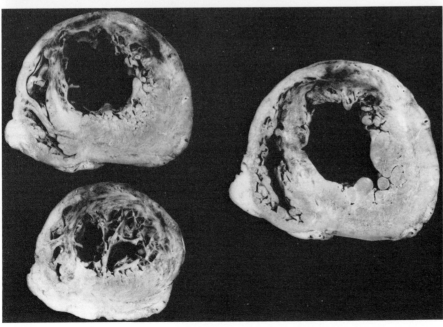

Fig. 11. Cross-section of ventricles showing a zone of discoloration and thinning of the anteroseptal segment of the LV 10 days after acute infarction. Fig. 11 used with permission of Springer-Verlag New York Inc. from Coronary Heart Disease, Clinical, Angiographic and Pathologic Profile, 1976 by Vlodaver Z., Amplatz K., Burchell H. B. and Edwards J. E.

B. Anatomic Locations of Infarction

2. Anterobasal Infarction

Located in the anterior wall of the LV, including the anterior half of the anterolateral papillary muscle, and may include the septum, slices 4 and 5.

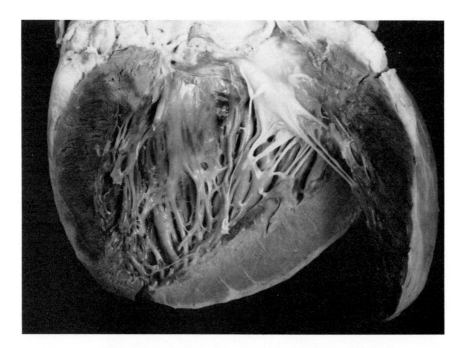

Fig. 12. Left ventricle from inside. There is an extensive infarction involving the apical and base portion of the anteroseptal region of the LV, characterized by discoloration of the wall. Fig. 12 used with permission of Springer-Verlag New York Inc. from Coronary Heart Disease, Clinical, Angiographic and Pathologic Profile, 1976 by Vlodaver Z., Amplatz K., Burchell H. B. and Edwards J. E.

B. Anatomic Locations of Infarction

3. Anterolateral Infarction

Involves the anteroseptal and lateral wall of the LV, extending from slice 1 to 4.

4. Lateral Infarction

Located in the lateral wall of the LV, between the anterior edge of the posteromedial papillary muscle and the middle of the anterolateral papillary muscle, slices 2 to 4.

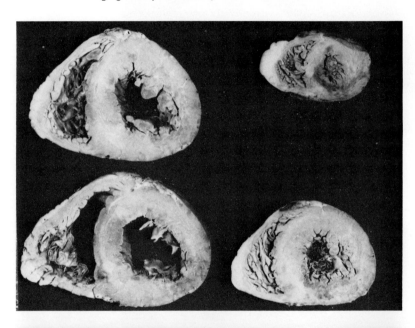

Fig. 13. Cross-section of ventricles, demonstrating discoloration of the lateral wall of the LV one day after acute infarction. Fig. 13 used with permission of Springer-Verlag New York Inc. from Coronary Heart Disease, Clinical, Angiographic and Pathologic Profile, 1976 by Vlodaver Z., Amplatz K., Burchell H. B. and Edwards J. E.

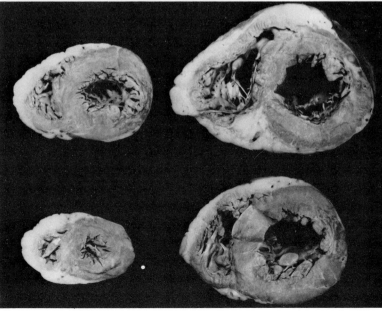

Fig. 14. Cross-section of the ventricular portion of the heart three weeks following acute myocardial lateral infarction. This shows thinning involving the lateral wall of the LV including the anterolateral papillary muscle. Fig. 14 used with permission of Springer-Verlag New York Inc. from Coronary Heart Disease, Clinical, Angiographic and Pathologic Profile, 1976 by Vlodaver Z., Amplatz K., Burchell H. B. and Edwards J. E.

B. Anatomic Locations of Infarction

9. Septal Infarction
Involves the IV septum.

10. Apical Infarction
Involves the LV apex only. May be anterior, lateral, inferior or circumferential, slices 1 and 2.

11. Circumferential infarction
Extends over the anteroposterior, lateral and septal walls of the LV.

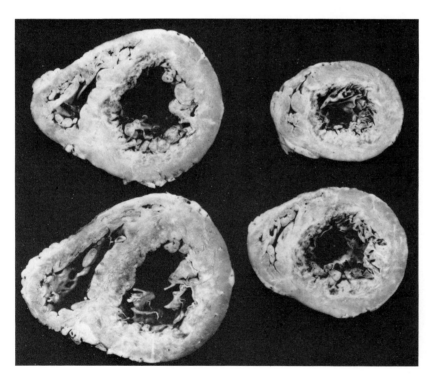

Fig. 17. Cross-section of ventricles, with a circumferential healed infarction. Fig. 17 used with permission of Springer-Verlag New York Inc. from Coronary Heart Disease, Clinical, Angiographic and Pathologic Profile, 1976 by Vlodaver Z., Amplatz K., Burchell H. B. and Edwards J. E.

Two-dimensional echocardiography shows asynergy in more than two-thirds of the segments where myocardial infarction was seen in autopsy.

In correlated pathological studies, the estimation of asynergia exceeds the size of the infarct. This finding suggests that the area of asynergia may include a myocardium with some degree of reversible injury.

C. M-Mode Echocardiographic Patterns

M-mode echocardiography may detect wall motion abnormalities, left ventricular dilatation and myocardial scarring as results of myocardial infarction.

Acute myocardial ischemia will result in alterations of the contraction pattern, represented on the M-mode echocardiogram as reduced systolic amplitude and velocity of motion, and a decreased systolic thickening.

Normal septum motion amplitude ranges from 5 to 8 mm and inferior wall amplitude, from 8 to 12 mm.

Normal thickening of the IV septum during systolic contraction is more than 30% and for the inferior wall more than 45%.

Direct visualization of segmental wall motion abnormalities is represented by hypokinesis, akinesis and dyskinesis of segments of the LV wall, and these are good indicators of myocardium affected by ischemia and/or scarring.

Non-ischemic segments of the LV may demonstrate exaggerated amplitude of motion as a compensatory phenomenon.

Scarring of the LV wall is classically recognized as increased wall density, decreased motion and reduced thickness, and usually measures 7 mm or less. The limitation of M-mode study is that it allows analysis only of the basal and mid portion of the LV wall, so the apical portion of the LV is inaccesible to analysis.

Left Ventricular Function: The end-diastolic LV internal dimension is a good indicator of LV size.

Velocity of circumferential (fractional) shortening (mean VCF) is an important index of LV function that takes into account the velocity of LV wall motion and the extent of shortening, and reduced values indicate decreased contractility of the LV wall. Another useful index is the ejection fraction (EF), expressed in percent and calculated as stroke volume/end diastolic ventricular volume.

C. M-Mode Echocardiographic Patterns

Delayed closure of the mitral valve (prolonged AC interval) interrupted by a "B" notch indicates elevated end-diastolic pressure.

Monitoring the LV function indices and chamber dimensions by serial studies, and sequential changes in these variables may provide a sensitive noninvasive method of detecting cardiac enlargement, ventricular dysfunction or a functional response to therapeutic approaches in the individual patient with acute myocardial infarction.

C. M-Mode Echocardiographic Patterns

1. Anterior Wall Infarction

Patients with acute anterior wall infarction have abnormally decreased septal motion, abnormally reduced septal systolic thickening, and systolic thinning of the interventricular septum. Akinesis and paradoxical septal wall motion are frequent findings in patients with anterior infarction.

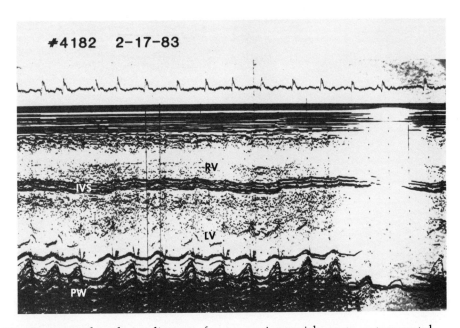

Fig. 18. M-mode echocardiogram from a patient with acute anteroseptal myocardial infarction. The amplitude of the interventricular septal motion and its systolic thickening are reduced. The septum is relatively echo-dense compared with the posterior wall and is thin in diastole. The motion of the posterior wall is increased, to compensate for the poor motion of the interventricular septum.

C. M-Mode Echocardiographic Patterns

2. Anteroseptal Infarction

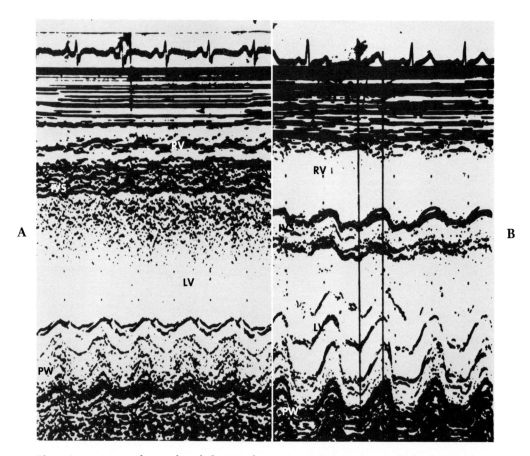

Fig. 19. A, M-mode study of the LV from a patient with acute transmural anteroseptal infarction, showing akinesis of the interventricular septum, enlarged left ventricle. **B,** LV echocardiogram showing dyskinesis of the interventricular septum from a patient who developed an anteroseptal infarction following coronary bypass surgery.

C. M-Mode Echocardiographic Patterns

3. Inferior Wall Infarction

Patients with acute inferior infarction have abnormally reduced posterior wall thickening and decreased posterior wall motion.

Paradoxical wall motion and systolic thinning of the posterior wall are less frequently recorded with inferior infarction.

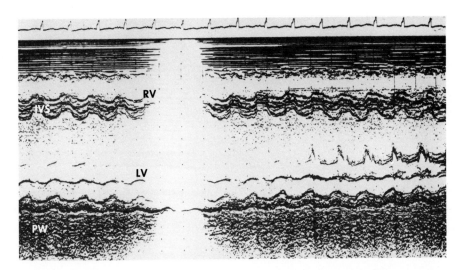

Fig. 20. M-mode echocardiogram from a patient with acute inferior wall myocardial infarction. The amplitude of the left ventricular posterior wall motion and its systolic thickening are diminished. There is hyperactivity of the interventricular septum, as compensation for the poor posterior wall motion.

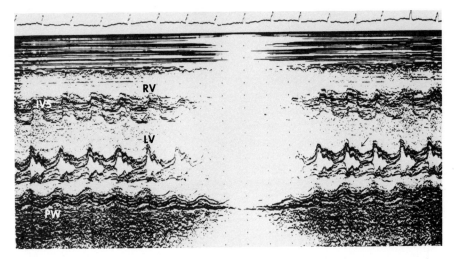

Fig. 21. Mitral valve from the same patient in fig. 20 with extensive inferior wall infarction, showing prolonged A-C interval and "B" notch (arrow) associated with elevated end-diastolic pressure. Very small pericardial effusion. LVEF 30%.

C. M-Mode Echocardiographic Patterns

3. Inferior Wall Infarction

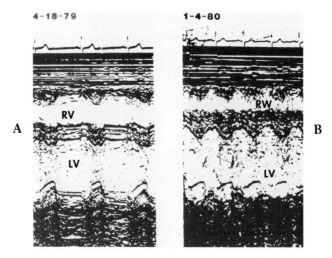

Fig. 22. A, LV echocardiogram of a patient with angina, one year prior to infarction, showing normal motion of the interventricular septum and the inferior wall. **B,** LV echocardiogram from the same patient one year later following acute myocardial infarction of the inferior wall, showing hypokinesis and reduced systolic thickening of the inferior wall.

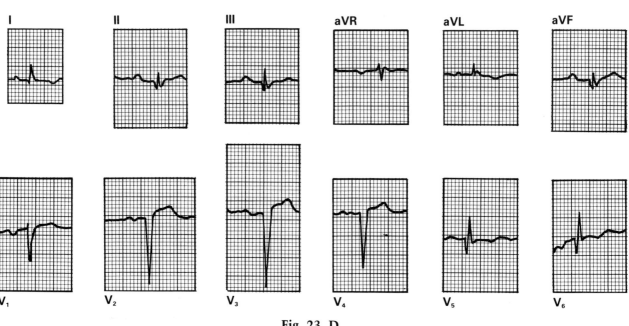

Fig. 23. D

C. M-Mode Echocardiographic Patterns

Shown on this page is an LV echocardiogram from a patient with recent anteroseptal infarction, and an old healed inferior wall infarction demonstrating the limitation of M-mode study to analyze the apical portion of the LV.

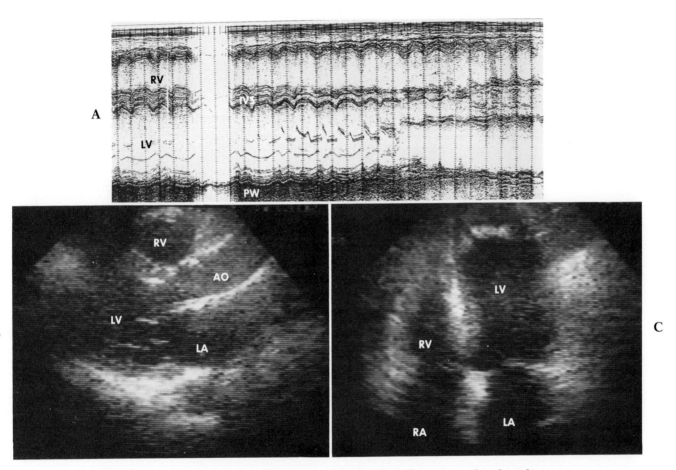

Fig. 23. A, M-Mode echocardiogram showing hypokinesis and reduced systolic thickening of the inferior wall. The motion pattern of the IV septum appears normal. **B,** Parasternal long axis view of the same patient showing thinning of the inferior wall. **C,** Apical four-chamber view, showing dilatation of the apical segment of the LV, with thinning of the wall, and in real time appears akinetic. These findings are compatible with the recent anteroseptal infarction. Mass of dense echoes in the apical portion of the LV, compatible with apical thrombus. **D,** (see opposite page) ECG three days after admission showing feature characteristics of inferior and anteroseptal infarction, first degree of A-V block.

D. Two-Dimensional Echocardiographic Evaluation

Two-dimensional echocardiography permits the evaluation of anatomic location, extent and severity of acute infarction.

Two-dimensional echocardiography offers the ability to evaluate segmental abnormalities with much greater facility than M-mode examination since the field of the examination is not restricted to the narrow M-mode beam.

Special orientation allows analysis of all wall segments, often with multiple views of the same segment. In most of the cases with acute myocardial infarction over a time of 24 hours, wall motion abnormalities occur.

Segmental wall motion and contraction abnormalities (asynergia) are characterized by a decreased amplitude of endocardial excursion and decreased wall thickening of the infarcted myocardium. This may be visually identified by comparing with adjacent normally moving segments.

With adequate study, segmental abnormal motion can be demonstrated in all the cases with transmural infarction.

With focal or subendocardial infarction, abnormal wall motion can not be detected in some patients.

Abnormal wall motion is classified as: *Hypokinetic,* when there is reduced motion and decreased systolic thickening of the infarcted segment.

Akinetic: When there is absence of motion and systolic thickening of the wall.

Dyskinetic or *Paradoxic:* When there is systolic endocardial expansion and thinning of the wall.

Myocardial scarring following acute myocardial infarction is recognized by an increase in density, and thinning of the infarcted segment.

The area of asynergia usually will not vary in the first 3 to 4 days of the acute infarction, but after this period of time, extension of this area of asynergia may occur and be identified with two-dimensional echocardiographic studies.

D. Two-Dimensional Echocardiographic Evaluation

Extension of the infarcted segment may be clinically silent.

Expansion of the infarcted area a few days after the infarction is recognized by thinning of the wall and enlargement of the area of asynergia, and is indicative of transmural infarction.

Patients with anterior and anteroseptal infarction seem particularly prone to expansion of the infarcted area.

Two-dimensional echocardiography can be used as an indicator of segmental changes that occur in the evolution of patients with acute myocardial infarction and has significant clinical value in assessing interventions and prognosis for such patients.

D. Two-Dimensional Echocardiographic Evaluation

1. Anteroseptal Infarction

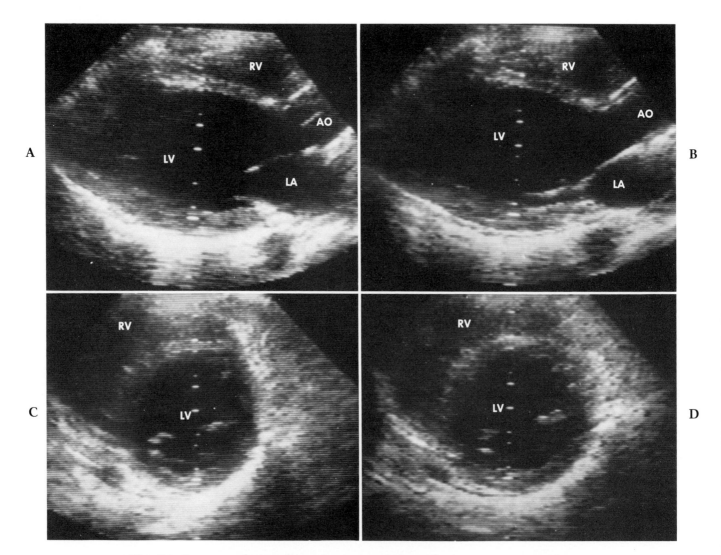

Fig. 24. Parasternal recordings from a patient with acute anteroseptal infarction three days following admission. The interventricular septum and anterior wall motion is hypokinetic, and the systolic thickening reduced; the LV function values are reduced. Parasternal long axis view: **A,** Diastole; **B,** Systole. Parasternal short axis view: **C,** Diastole; and **D,** Systole.

D. Two-Dimensional Echocardiographic Evaluation

1. *Anteroseptal Infarction:*

Shown on this and the next page are illustrations from a patient with a past history of angina and recent anteroseptal infarction.

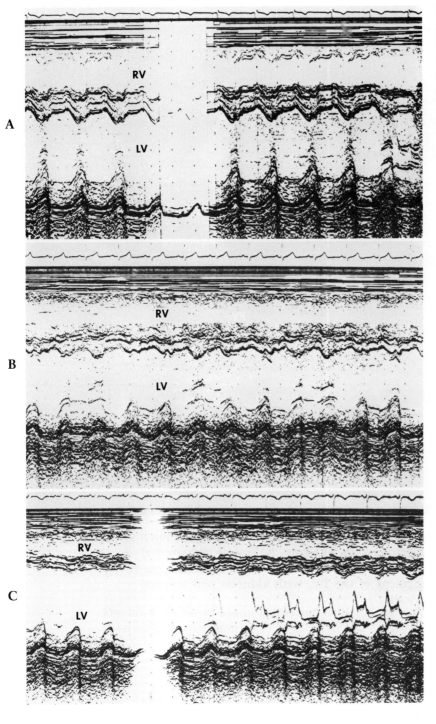

Fig. 25. M-mode LV echocardiogram study from a patient with angina (**A** and **B**) two and three years prior to infarction, showing normal motion and systolic thickening of the IV septum and inferior wall. **C**, LV echocardiogram from the same patient, one week after the infarction. The IVS motion and systolic thickening are reduced.

D. Two-Dimensional Echocardiographic Evaluation

4. Acute Inferior Wall Infarction

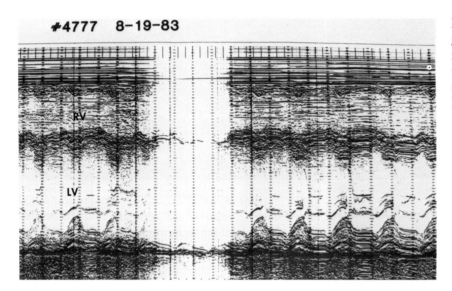

Fig. 34. M-Mode LV echocardiogram from a patient with acute inferior wall infarction, as illustrated on the previous page, shows adequate motion of the IVS and PW.

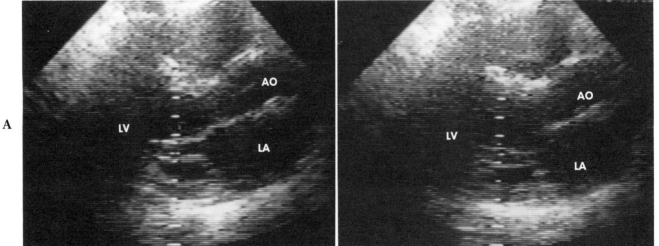

Fig. 35. Two-dimensional echocardiogram from the same patient shown in figure 34. Parasternal long axis view in diastole (**A**) and systole (**B**), demonstrates thinning and reduced systolic thickening of the inferobasal segment of the LV, beneath the posterior leaflet of the mitral valve. and hypokinesis of this segment in real time.

D. Two-Dimensional Echocardiographic Evaluation

5. Apical Lateral Infarction

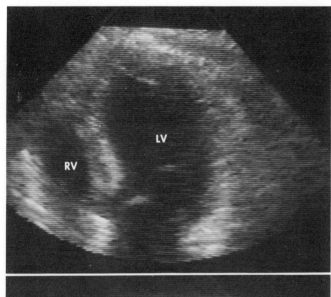

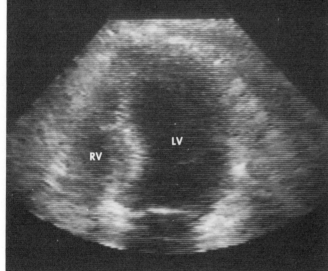

Fig. 36. Apical four-chamber view, in diastole (**A**) and systole (**B**), showing thinning and reduced systolic thickening of the apical lateral segment of the LV, 5 days after admission for acute infarction. The ECG revealed Q waves and ST-T segmental changes in leads Li, aVL and pronounced inverted T waves in precordial leads.

D. Two-Dimensional Echocardiographic Evaluation

6. *Right ventricular infarction*

Right ventricular infarction may occur as an extension of inferior wall infarction of the LV.

The echocardiographic features include RV wall abnormalities; akinesis or dyskinesis of the diaphragmatic wall of the RV; signs of RV volume overload: enlargement of the RV, paradoxical ventricular septal wall motion and tricuspid insufficiency.

Shown in figure 37 **A** to **D,** illustrations from a patient with acute infarction of the RV, complicating inferobasal and posteroseptal infarction of the LV; and new murmur of tricuspid insufficiency.

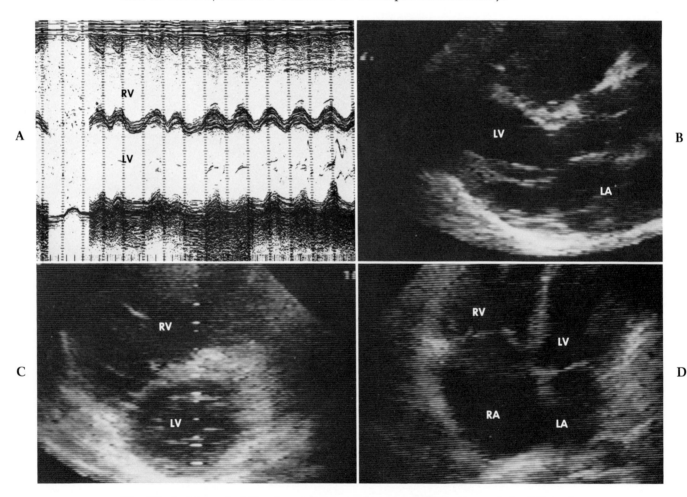

Fig. 37. A, M-mode LV echocardiogram showing enlargement of the RV and paradoxical motion of the IV septum. **B,** Two-dimensional echocardiogram, parasternal long axis view, showing dilatation of the inferobasal segment of the LV, with thinning of the wall and akinesis in real time. **C,** Parasternal short axis view, showing thinning of the posteroseptal segment of the IVS and in real time akinesis of the posterior wall of the RV. **D,** Apical four-chamber view showing enlargement of the RV and RA and in real time signs of RV volume overload.

D. Two-Dimensional Echocardiographic Evaluation

7. Circumferential Infarction

Shown on this page are LV echocardiograms from a patient with acute infarction of the anteroseptal and inferolateral segments of the LV apex, called circumferential infarction.

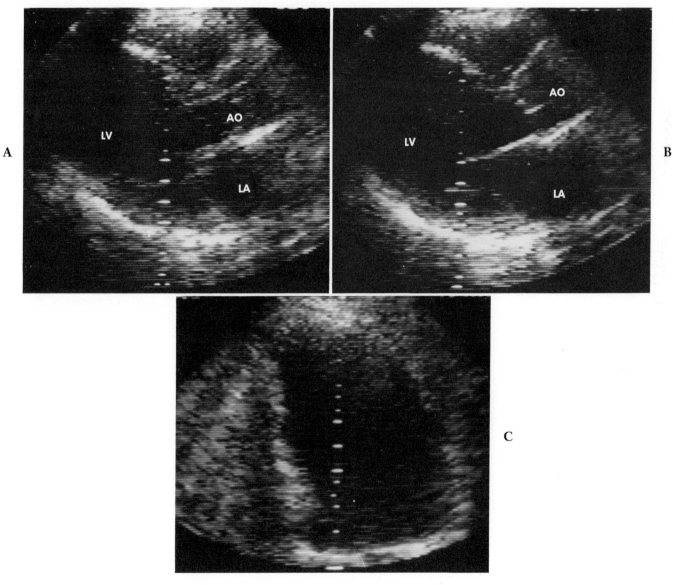

Fig. 38. Parasternal long axis view showing thinning and poor systolic thickening of the IVS. **A,** Systole. **B,** Diastole. **C,** Apical two-chamber view, showing dilated apical segment of the LV, with reduced systolic thickening of the anteroseptal and lateral segments.

E. ECG Correlation

1. *With Pathologic Findings*

Most reports correlating electrocardiographic and pathologic findings in acute myocardial infarction agree that the electrocardiographic diagnosis is usually correct. However, the electrocardiogram is generally less precise in diagnosis and localization of healed myocardial infarction.

The electrocardiogram underestimates the extent of a myocardial infarction. When a healed myocardial infarct at a specific location is recognized by electrocardiographic criteria, it is likely that there are unrecognized infarcts involving other areas of the left ventricle.

Infarction involving the lateral and inferobasal areas are frequently unrecognized.

Apical myocardial infarction does not appear to have specific electrocardiographic findings, other than those related to general infarct localization by electrocardiogram, particularly in patients with anteroseptal or anterolateral infarction.

Abnormal Q waves, generally thought to indicate transmural infarction, are frequently found in subendocardial infarction.

E. ECG Correlation

2. With M-Mode LV Echocardiogram

Abnormal motion and contraction patterns of the left ventricular wall as recorded with M-mode study correspond to the ECG site of an infarction in most cases of anteroseptal and/or inferior wall infarction. See table in Figure 39.

There is no good correlation to identified lateral wall injury.

Infarction of the apical portion of the left ventricle is poorly reflected in the M-mode studies.

ECG-ECHO CORRELATION

TOTAL 48 CASES	ACUTE MI	ABNORMAL LV PATTERN
25	ANTERIOR	24 IVS MOTION ↓ △% ↓ 1 PW MOTION ↓ △% ↓
22	INFERIOR	22 PW MOTION ↓ △% ↓
3	LATERAL	2 PW MOTION ↓ △% ↓ 1 IVS MOTION ↓ △% ↓

Fig. 39. Shows correlation of ECG and abnormal LV M-mode patterns in a group of 48 patients with acute myocardial infarction.

E. ECG Correlation

3. *With Two-Dimensional Echocardiogram*

Two-dimensional echocardiogram is a better predictor of the extent and location of the acute infarction.

95% of the patients with electrocardiographic evidence of infarction involving the *inferior wall* (Q waves in leads 2,3 aVF) will have abnormal wall motion involving the inferior or inferoposterior wall of the left ventricle.

When the abnormal motion of the inferior wall is associated with acute infarction of the interventricular septum, with rupture or aneurysm of the septum, it is not indicated by the electrocardiogram in most of the cases.

Most patients with ECG changes consistent with acute *anterior infarction* will show abnormal motion and contraction patterns of the anterior wall at the mid ventricular level. In patients with an ECG diagnosis of anteroseptal infarction, abnormal motion occurs in the anterior wall and interventricular septum at the mid ventricle, with involvement of the cardiac apex.

The apical dysfunction is poorly reflected electrocardiographically.

The anterobasal portion of the LV is less frequently involved, and abnormalities in the motion of this segment imply extensive and severe myocardial infarction. Clinical and ECG evidence of subendocardial, or focal, infarction may not be reflected or recognized in the echocardiogram early recordings; in such cases, a repeat study a few days after the heart attack, or a followup study, may detect the abnormal motion of the segment involved by the injury.

In patients with electrocardiographic diagnosis of acute *lateral infarction*, the abnormalities in the motion of the lateral wall occur in the mid segment of the left ventricle.

In most cases, infarction of the lateral wall is associated with either infarction in the inferior wall or anterior wall. With inferolateral infarction, the abnormal motion of the lateral wall involves the base of the left ventricle. With anterolateral infarction, the lateral segment of the mid ventricle and the apical portion of the LV, uniformly show abnormal motion.

E. ECG Correlation

3. With Two-Dimensional Echocardiogram

Two-dimensional LV echocardiogram can show segmental abnormality of motion and contraction pattern of the infarcted area within 24 hours of initial event in most cases with acute infarction.

Early performance of echocardiography in patients admitted to CCU to rule out MI will help make and exclude diagnosis of infarction in cases with non-diagnostic ECG. LBBB, or other intraventricular conduction, defects and with non-specific ST-T changes.

SECTION III

ECHOCARDIOGRAPHIC RECOGNITION OF COMPLICATIONS

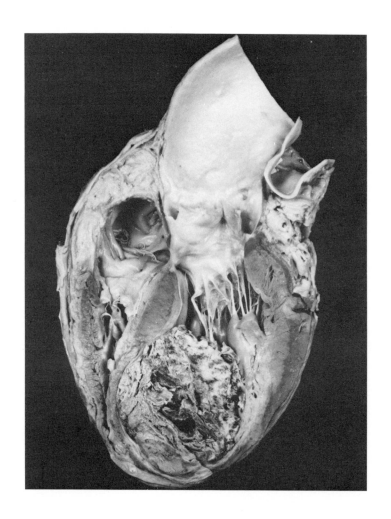

A. Definition

Severe complications of acute myocardial infarction usually are cardiac, and classified either as arrhythmias or heart failure ("pump failure").

Severe ventricular arrhythmias, ventricular tachycardia or ventricular fibrillation, may lead to the death of patients with acute myocardial infarction, and usually are preceded by ventricular ectopic or premature beats.

Acute heart failure is related to severe impairment of LV function and, in general, to an extensive amount of myocardial damage. It is less commonly related to mitral insufficiency, acquired left-to-right shunt, or an aneurysm complicating the myocardial infarction.

Clinically, in its final stages, pump failure is manifested as shock (hypotension) dyspnea and pulmonary edema.

Extracardiac complications of acute myocardial infarction are less common, and include systemic thromboembolism from an intracardiac thrombus.

B. Pericardial Effusion

Pericarditis is a complication in cases with transmural infarction, usually detected within 4 to 5 days after the infarction. It is often unrecognized in spite of typical chest pain, because of the absence of a pericardial rub or ECG changes, and in many cases is first detected by echocardiographic studies.

Typical symptoms are recurrent chest pain, aggravated by deep inspiration or change of position; dyspnea and low-grade fever. Friction rub in the precordium is present. Recurrence may occur a few weeks later: postmyocardial infarction or Dressler Syndrome. The cause is unknown, but it has been attributed to a hypersensitivity reaction in which the antigen is the necrotic myocardium.

At times pericarditis is the dominant finding preceding rupture of the heart and cardiac tamponade.

Echocardiography is a sensitive technique for evaluation of patients with pericardial effusion.

Moderate pericardial effusion is defined as effusion that creates an anterior and posterior echo-free space between the epicardium and pericardium and is present in systole.

Large pericardial effusion is defined as effusion large enough to allow visible swinging of the heart within the pericardial space.

Cardiac tamponade is the hemodynamic consequence of an increase in intrapericardial pressure that equals or exceeds the normal filling pressure of the right ventricle and the left ventricle, with subsequent reduced right ventricular filling, and decline in cardiac output and blood pressure.

Clinically cardiac tamponade is recognized by the presence of moderate to large pericardial effusion, associated with elevated venous pressure, hypotension (systolic arterial pressure less than 100mm Hg), and pulsus paradoxus at least 10mmHg.

B. Pericardial Effusion

M-mode signs include right ventricular compression, respiratory variations in left ventricular and right ventricular dimension, and abnormalities in mitral valve motion. Abnormal right ventricular wall motion includes posterior movement of the right ventricular free wall in early and mid diastole, as timed with electrocardiogram monitoring.

Two-dimensional echocardiography will reveal abnormal right ventricular wall motion as an indentation of the right ventricular free wall during early diastole. This posterior motion of the right ventricular free wall in diastole represents a true collapse of the right ventricle and indicates that intrapericardial pressure is elevated and approaches or exceeds the filling pressure of the right ventricle.

B. Pericardial Effusion

The following illustrations are from a patient with acute infero-lateral infarction, with recurrent chest pain, fever and a friction rub in the chest on auscultation, on the 10th day after his infarction (Dressler Syndrome).

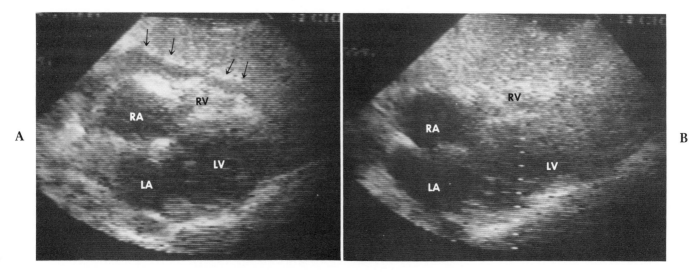

Fig. 40. Subxiphoid four-chamber view: **A,** Small pericardial effusion (arrows). **B,** No effusion seen after treatment with salycilates.

B. Pericardial Effusion

The following are illustrations from a patient with large pericardial effusion, swinging of the heart, and signs of cardiac tamponade.

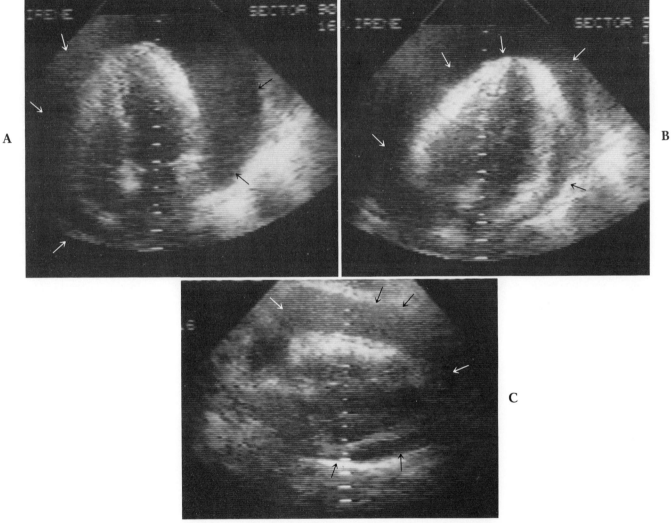

Fig. 41. Apical four-chamber view: Apex pointing to the right (**A**) and to the left (**B**) during diastole and systole respectively. Large free space of 30mm shows in the anterior and posterior aspects of the pericardium. **C,** Subxiphoid four-chamber view with large effusion. The anterior wall of the RV shows an indentation during early diastole, as seen with tamponade. Arrows: pericardial effusion.

C. Heart ("Pump") Failure with Extensive Myocardial Damage

In cases with recent myocardial infarction and heart failure, the type of infarction is usually transmural.

Heart failure may also result from an acute subendocardial injury, plus extensive damage from a previously healed infarction.

Congestive heart failure following myocardial infarction implies failure of both ventricles, with increased pulmonary and systemic venous pressure. There is a low cardiac output and retention of salt and water.

C. Heart ("Pump") Failure with Extensive Myocardial Damage

1. Congestive Heart Failure

Cardiac function is governed by the integration of four determinants of cardiac output: preload—the venous return to the heart or end-diastolic volume of the ventricle; afterload—the tension developed by the ventricle, a function of intraventricular volume and systolic pressure; contractility and rhythm. Alteration of any determinant may cause heart failure. In acute myocardial infarction congestive heart failure occurs because of impairment in cardiac contractility, usually related to extensive damage with significant reduction in the cardiac output.

The kidneys respond to low cardiac output, with retention of sodium and water. Further expansion in the vascular volume (hypervolemia) leads to activation of the renin-angiotensin-aldosterone system. Hypervolemia, in turn, leads to an increase in the venous return to the heart (increase in the preload) and an increase in the volume and size of the LV (increase in afterload).

Hypervolemia in congestive heart failure leads to inappropriate elevation in systemic vascular resistance (due to elevated levels of circulating catecholamines, increase in sympathetic vasoconstrictor tone and increase in vascular stiffness because of expansion of vascular volume). This elevated systemic vascular resistance results in further increase of arterial pressure and LV afterload. Treatment of congestive heart failure and its clinical manifestation of pulmonary congestion and peripheral edema involve the use of a digitalis glycoside to increase the contractile force of the heart, diuretics to reduce the circulatory volume, and reduction of preload and aftermath with systemic vasodilator drugs. This approach has become the most important advance in therapy.

E. Left Ventricular Aneurysm

True LV aneurysm is characterized by thinning of the cardiac wall in the infarcted area, with "bulging" of the external contour.

The wall of the aneurysm is comprised of muscle fibers and scar tissue. With time, fibrosis and calcified changes are the predominant components of the wall of the aneurysm.

Formation of thrombi in a ventricular aneurysm and subsequent systemic embolisms are commom complications. Serious ventricular arrhythmias and congestive heart failure are commonly associated with LV aneurysm. Rupture of the wall of a true aneurysm is a rare complication. It may occur in 5 to 15% of the cases with prior transmural infarction. In 95% of the cases, the LV aneurysms are anteroapical; the remaining are inferobasal or inferoseptal. Palpation of the precordium gives us a sustained or double impulse. On auscultation, a third and fourth sound are common. The electrocardiogram shows persistent ST-T segmental elevation and, on x-ray, a localized bulging of the LV with calcified changes is an important sign.

M-mode echocardiography is useful in the detection of LV aneurysms in only 50% of the cases with angiographically proved LV aneurysms.

In the standard M-mode examination, a scan of the LV from the base to apex will show that the cavity expands, or fails to be recorded, as the region of the papillary muscle is approached.

Two-dimensional echocardiography permits the detection of an LV aneurysm with accuracy in 90 to 100% of the cases (sensitivity in 93% and specificity in 84%). The echocardiographic appearance of a true aneurysm is one of a demarcated bulge of the LV, both in systole and diastole, with thinning of the wall. The motion is paradoxic and the aneurysm has a wide neck, the diameter being comparable to the diameter of the aneurysm.

E. Left Ventricular Aneurysm

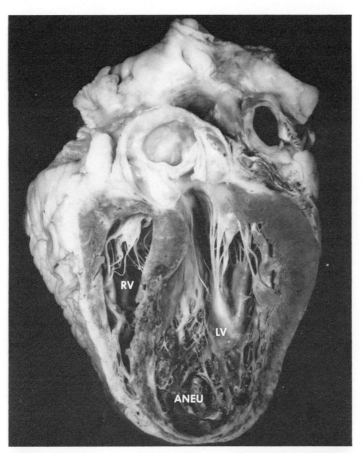

Fig. 45. Frontal section of the heart showing a true aneurysm of the anteroseptal portion of the LV. The interventricular septum and apical walls are thin and show an aneurysmal bulge. A small thrombus has formed in the cavity. One of the features of a true ventricular aneurysm is a wide neck leading to the fundus. Fig. 45 used with permission of Springer-Verlag New York Inc. from Coronary Heart Disease, Clinical, Angiographic and Pathologic Profile, 1976 by Vlodaver Z., Amplatz K., Burchell H. B. and Edwards J. E.

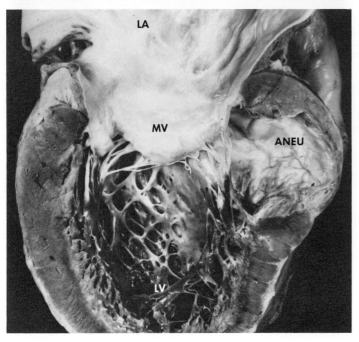

Fig. 46. Left ventricular aneurysm of the inferior type from inside the LV, showing a bulge in the posterobasal region of the LV. The aneurysm has a wide neck connecting to and communicating with the LV cavity, the wall is thin and is associated with infarction of the papillary muscle.

E. Left Ventricular Aneurysm

Shown on this and the next page are illustrations from a patient with transmural anteroseptal infarction and LV apical aneurysm.

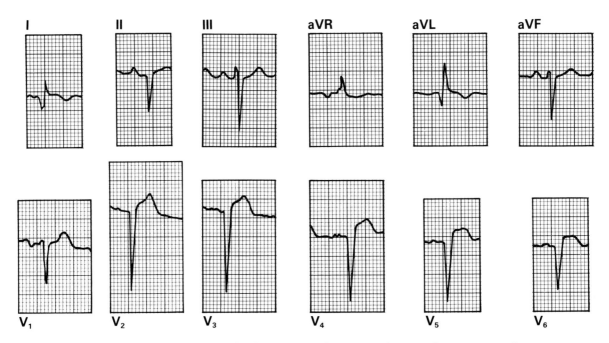

Fig. 47. A, ECG—Day of admission. Classic evidence of anteroseptal myocardial infarction and additional signs, particularly Q waves in leads I and aLV, of involvement of the lateral wall.

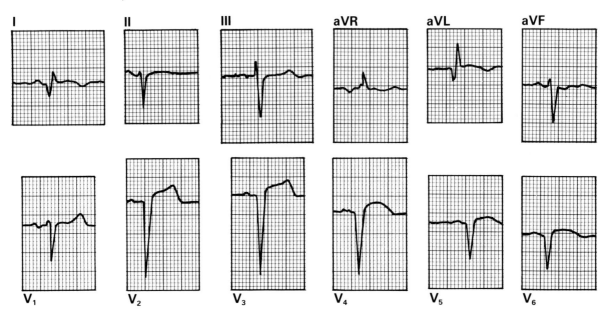

Fig. 47. B, Persistence of elevated ST segments in the precordial leads is consistent with an LV anterior apical aneurysm.

E. Left Ventricular Aneurysm

The following two-dimensional echocardiograms are from the patient with transmural anteroseptal infarction and LV apical aneurysm, whose ECG tracings are shown on the previous page.

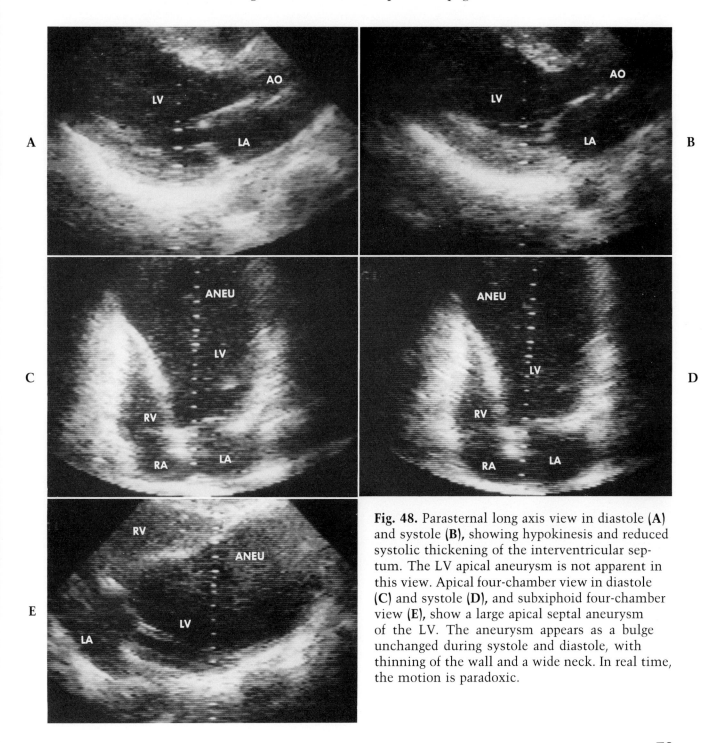

Fig. 48. Parasternal long axis view in diastole (**A**) and systole (**B**), showing hypokinesis and reduced systolic thickening of the interventricular septum. The LV apical aneurysm is not apparent in this view. Apical four-chamber view in diastole (**C**) and systole (**D**), and subxiphoid four-chamber view (**E**), show a large apical septal aneurysm of the LV. The aneurysm appears as a bulge unchanged during systole and diastole, with thinning of the wall and a wide neck. In real time, the motion is paradoxic.

E. Left Ventricular Aneurysm

Shown on this page are two-dimensional recordings from a patient with anteroseptal infarction complicated with small apical aneurysm.

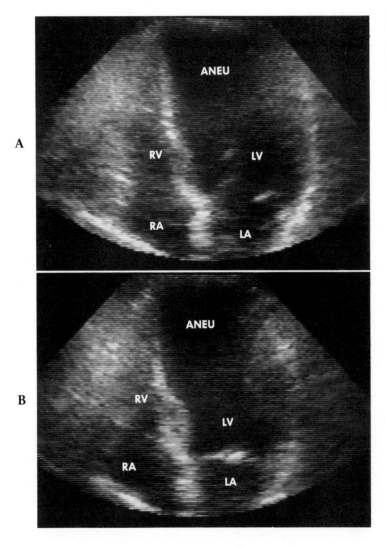

Fig. 49. Apical four-chamber view. **A,** Diastole. **B,** Systole, showing localized dilatation of the apical portion of the LV, with thinning of the wall, and deviation of the apical segment of the IV septum to the right. In real time, the motion is paradoxic.

E. Left Ventricular Aneurysm

Illustrations from a patient with inferior wall infarction and aneurysm of the inferobasal segment of the LV.

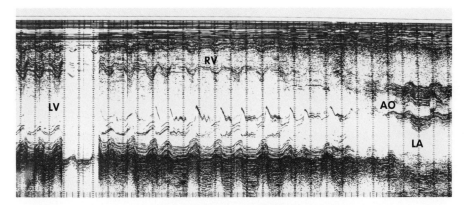

Fig. 50. M-mode LV echocardiogram showing hypokinesis and reduced systolic thickening of the PW. The LV is enlarged and the LV function values reduced. In most of the cases, the inferior aneurysm cannot be identified by M-mode echocardiography.

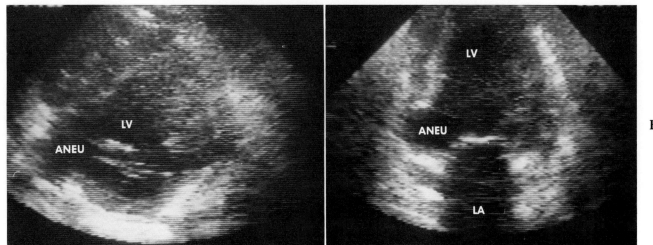

Fig. 51. A, Short axis view. **B,** Apical two-chamber view. The aneurysm appears as bulging of the inferior wall, with thinning of the wall.

E. Left Ventricular Aneurysm

Inferoseptal aneurysm is not uncommon, and follows myocardial infarction of the inferior wall and proximal segment of the interventricular septum.

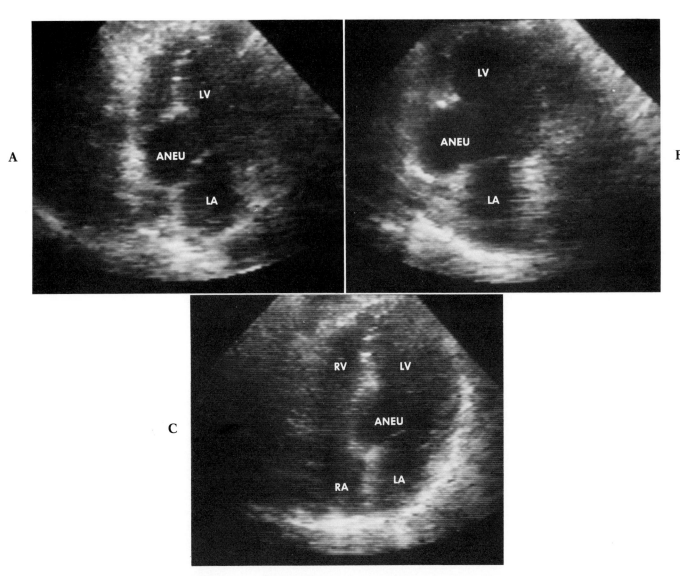

Fig. 52. Apical two-chamber view in diastole (**A**) and systole (**B**), and apical four-chamber view (**C**) showing an inferoseptal aneurysm.

E. Left Ventricular Aneurysm

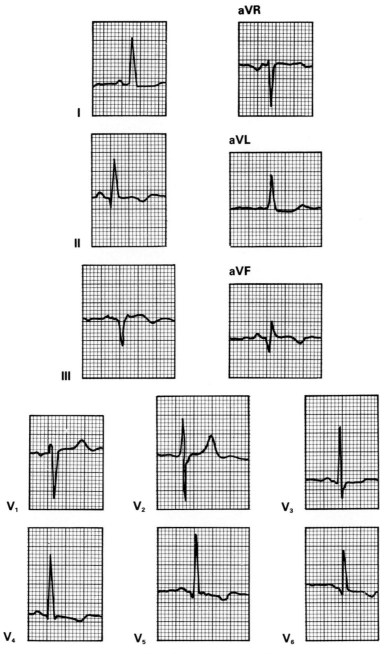

Fig. 53. ECG taken three weeks after admission showing a pattern of old inferior scar with persistence of ST segmental changes.

F. Intracardiac Thrombi

Thrombus formation occurs in about 17% of cases with acute myocardial infarction, more often with a transmural anterior wall, affecting the region of the cardiac apex, and frequently associated with left ventricular aneurysm.

Echocardiographic recognition of a thrombus is of clinical significance in the prevention of systemic arterial embolic events that occur in as many as 5% of patients following acute infarction.

Echocardiographically, a mural thrombus appears as a smooth, multilobular intracavitary mass that is contiguous with the ventricular wall in areas of akinesis or dyskinesis. Usually it is more echo-dense than the endocardium, and projects into the ventricular cavity.

An LV thrombus can be visualized as early as two days after the infarction, but more commonly in an average of five days after.

An apical thrombus is best visualized in the apical four-chamber view. The shape of the thrombus may be rounded-fixed, pedunculated, or broad-based, partially filling the cavity of an aneurysm, if present.

The false positive appearance of a thrombus may be related to artifacts, excessive trabeculation of the endocardium underlying scars or to a prominent papillary muscle.

F. Intracardiac Thrombi

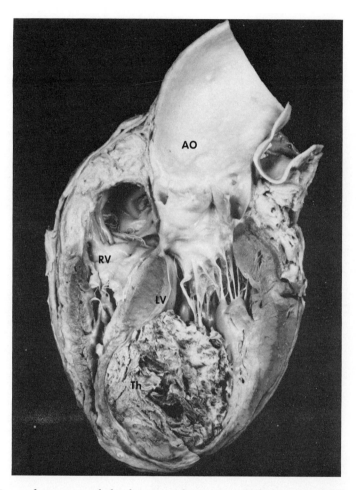

Fig. 54. Frontal section of the heart. A large rounded thrombus fills the cavity of a true aneurysm in the apical portion of the LV. Fig. 54 used with permission of Springer-Verlag New York Inc. from Coronary Heart Disease, Clinical, Angiographic and Pathologic Profile, 1976 by Vlodaver Z., Amplatz K., Burchell H. B. and Edwards J. E.

F. Intracardiac Thrombi

Shown on this and the next page are illustrations of cases with intracardiac thrombi of different shapes.

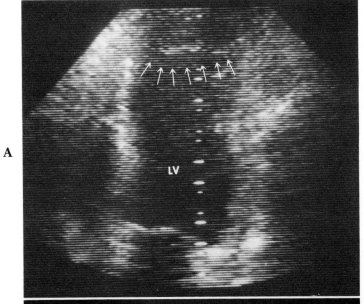

A

Fig. 55. A, Apical broad-based thrombus contiguous to area of akinesis. Apical four-chamber view. Arrows: thrombus.

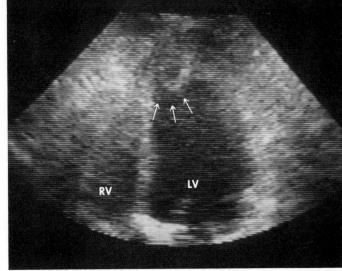

B

Fig. 55. B, Apical four-chamber view showing an apical "kidney shaped" thrombus from a patient with extensive anteroseptal infarction. Arrows: thrombus.

F. Intracardiac Thrombi

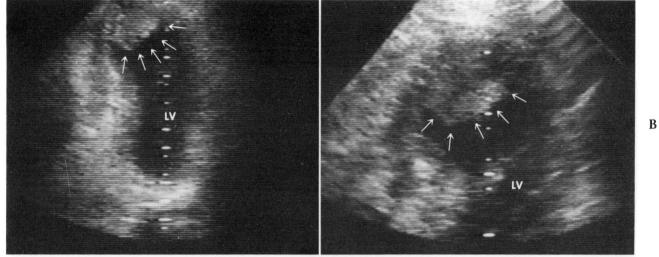

A   B

Fig. 56. Apical two-chamber view **(A)** and closeup view **(B)** of a large rounded thrombus (arrows) partially filling the cavity of an apical aneurysm.

G. Rupture of the Heart

Rupture of the heart is a relatively common complication among patients who die following acute myocardial infarction. This occurs in 10% of the cases, with the incidence greater among women.

Rupture occurs three to five days after the onset of the infarction and is usually transmural in nature.

The rupture occurs at the periphery of the infarction, near the non-infarcted myocardium. Rupture of the heart includes: rupture of the free wall of the LV, rupture of the ventricular septum and rupture of the papillary muscle.

G. Rupture of the Heart

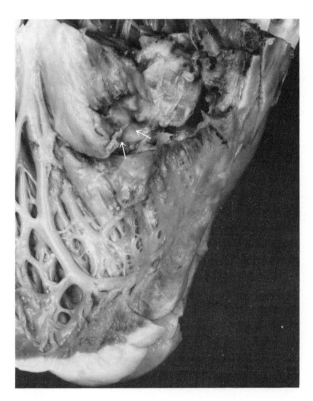

Fig. 62. Inside the LV there is a zone of discoloration and rupture tract into the ventricular septum (arrows) complicating acute transmural inferoseptal infarction. Fig. 62 used with permission by Springer-Verlag New York Inc. from Coronary Heart Disease, Clinical, Angiographic and Pathologic Profile, 1976 by Vlodaver Z., Amplatz K., Burchell H. B. and Edwards J. E.

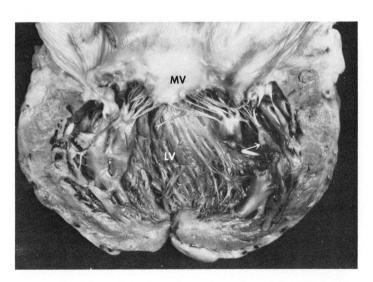

Fig. 63. Interior of the LV showing a classical rupture of the entire posteromedial papillary muscle complicating an acute transmural inferior wall infarction. Fig. 63 used with permission of the American Heart Association Inc. From Vlodaver Z. and Edwards J. E. Circulation 55:815, 1977.

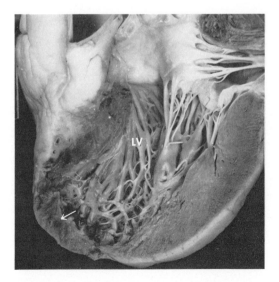

Fig. 64. Inside the LV, showing a rupture of the free wall at the apical segment of the LV complicating acute transmural anterior wall infarction (arrow). Fig. 64 used with permission of the American Heart Association Inc. From Vlodaver Z. and Edwards J. E. Circulation 55:815, 1977.

G. Rupture of the Heart

1. *Rupture of the Ventricular Septum*

Rupture of the ventricular septum is one of the significant, often catastrophic, complications of acute myocardial infarction, and constitutes 10% of all ruptures of the heart. In most of the cases with rupture of the interventricular septum, the infarction is transmural and antero-septal.

Clinically the condition is diagnosed when there is collapse of the circulation associated with a new murmur—holosystolic, loud, and maximal along the lower sternal border—most commonly between the second and third day after the onset of acute infarction. The association of the atrio-ventricular conduction defect occurs in 30% of the cases. Mortality occurs in 65% of the cases within two weeks and is related to a large shunt and severe progressive congestive heart failure.

When the ventricular septal defect is small, there is a better chance of survival and surgical closure of the defect.

Two-dimensional echocardiography permits direct visualization of the location of the septal perforation.

The defect appears as an interruption in the interventricular septum and is usually surrounded by areas of dyskinesis.

The size of the perforation may increase during systole as much as three times its diastolic diameter.

As a result of the acute left-to-right shunt, the left atrium and right ventricle will become enlarged and hyperkinesis (exaggerated motion) of the noninfarcted wall of the left ventricle will be present.

Peripherally venous injection of contrast material will confirm the presence of the shunt by displacement of the contrast material containing blood in the right ventricular cavity by the blood flowing from the left ventricle that does not contain the contrast material.

G. Rupture of the Heart

1. *Rupture of the Ventricular Septum*

M-mode echocardiographic findings in rupture of the ventricular septum are: dilatation of the right ventricle, unusual mitral valve movement with early closure of the valve, and abrupt posterior motion of the interventricular septum in early diastole. These findings are non-specific but their combination may be suggestive of rupture of the septum when associated with sudden appearance of a systolic murmur after acute myocardial infarction.

Two-dimensional echocardiographic findings in rupture of the ventricular septum may provide the size and location of the defect, usually in the muscular portion of the septum. Left-to-right shunt can be clearly recognized by detecting the jet of contrast-free left ventricular blood entering the contrast-filled right ventricle.

G. Rupture of the Heart

1. *Rupture of the Ventricular Septum*

Figures 65 and 66 are of a patient with acute anteroseptal infarction complicated by rupture of the ventricular septum and severe congestive heart failure.

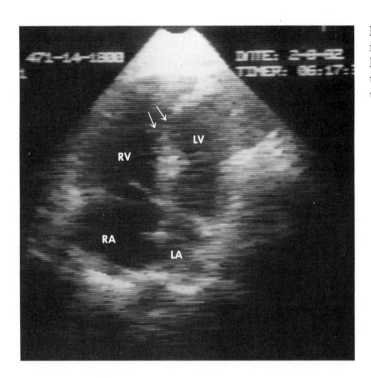

Fig. 65. Apical four-chamber view showing an interruption in the muscular portion of the IV septum (arrows) surrounded by areas of thinning of the wall, and dyskinesis in real time.

G. Rupture of the Heart

1. *Rupture of the Ventricular Septum*

Following rapid injection of contrast material into a peripheral vein, the presence of a shunt is confirmed by displacement of the contrast containing blood in the RV by the blood flowing from the LV.

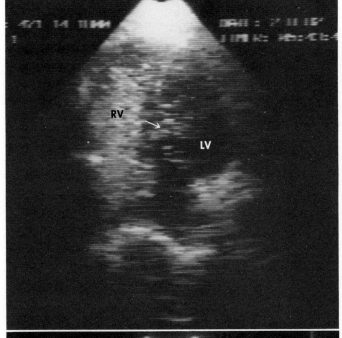

Fig. 66. A, Two-dimensional echocardiogram contrast study. Apical four-chamber view showing contrast material filling the RV and small amount going through the perforation into the LV cavity (arrow).

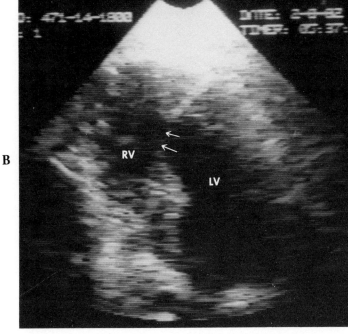

Fig. 66. B, Modified apical four-chamber view. Displacement of the contrast containing blood in the RV cavity by blood flowing from the LV at the site of the perforation (arrows).

G. Rupture of the Heart

2. *Rupture of the Papillary Muscle*

Rupture of the papillary muscle with mitral regurgitation accounts for about 1% of deaths from acute myocardial infarction, being less common than rupture of the free wall of the LV or of the ventricular septum.

Characteristically, rupture of the posteromedial papillary muscle occurs as a complication of inferior infarction.

Usually the entire muscle ruptures and the resulting mitral insufficiency is severe, causing early death. Less commonly, when rupture of a papillary muscle involves only a limited number of heads, mitral insufficiency is less severe and may be tolerated for months.

Characteristically, rupture of a papillary muscle is associated with a new systolic murmur, usually loud, apical, holosystolic, and diminishing before the second heart sound.

In those cases with sudden massive cardiac failure and cardiogenic shock, a murmur may be absent or may be obscured by the signs of pulmonary edema.

With M-mode study, rupture of the posterior papillary muscle and disruption of the mitral valve apparatus is represented by flail of the posterior leaflet.

The posterior mitral leaflet shows an abnormal motion during diastole characterized by chaotic and paradoxic motion, with coarse flutter, systolic left atrial echoes and systolic mitral valve prolapse.

When the anterior papillary muscle is the one disrupted, the common finding is an irregular motion of the anterior leaflet ("chaotic motion"), and the configuration changes from beat to beat.

Two-dimensional echocardiography allows clear visualization of papillary muscles and the mitral apparatus.

G. Rupture of the Heart

2. *Rupture of the Papillary Muscle*

Rupture of all or a portion of the papillary muscle produces a flail leaflet with prolapse of the chordal apparatus and valve tissue into the left atrium with each systole. Rupture of a papillary muscle producing severe mitral regurgitation is a surgically correctable problem. Average survival after papillary rupture is three days, which demonstrates the necessity for a prompt echocardiographic diagnosis and early surgical intervention.

G. Rupture of the Heart

2. *Rupture of the Papillary Muscle*
The following illustrations are from a patient with acute inferior wall infarction who developed congestive heart failure, hypotension and a new systolic murmur in the mitral area indicated on the fifth day following hospitalization. The clinical and echocardiographic findings indicated rupture of the papillary muscle of the mitral valve. Despite intensive care to stabilize his hemodynamic condition, the patient died the next day, before surgery could be performed.

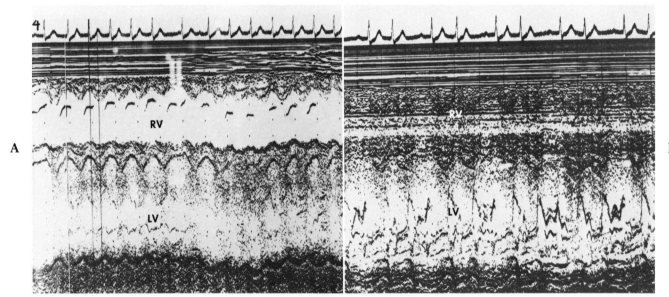

Fig. 67. M-mode echocardiogram from the patient with rupture of the papillary muscle of the mitral valve complicating acute inferior wall infarction. **A,** LV echocardiogram shows akinesis of the inferior wall and hyperkinetic IV septum. LV function reduced. **B,** Features of flail posterior mitral leaflet, coarse chaotic diastolic motion of the posterior mitral leaflet and initial paradoxic motion of the leaflet.

G. Rupture of the Heart

2. *Rupture of the Papillary Muscle*

Shown on this page is a partial rupture of the posteromedial papillary muscle in a patient with acute inferolateral infarction and a loud holosystolic murmur one week after the infarction.

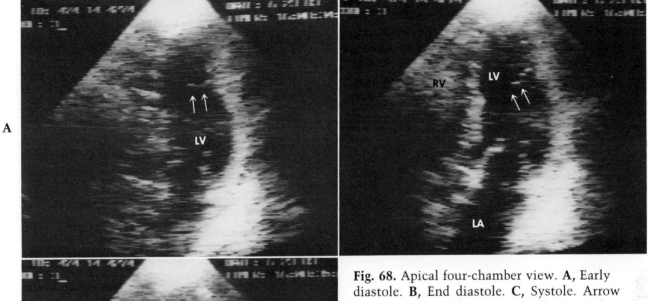

Fig. 68. Apical four-chamber view. **A,** Early diastole. **B,** End diastole. **C,** Systole. Arrow pointing to a portion of the papillary muscle with erratic motion. During systole bulging of the posterior leaflet clearly seen in real time.

A portion of one head of the posteromedial papillary muscle has ruptured incompletely, so that some continuity of the involved head is still present, and the characteristics of flail mitral valve are missing. Operation for severe mitral insufficiency was performed months after the onset of symptoms. During the operation partial rupture of the posteromedial papillary muscle was found and the mitral valve was replaced with a prosthesis.

G. Rupture of the Heart

3. *Rupture of the Free Wall and False Aneurysm*

Rupture of the free wall of the LV following myocardial infarction usually leads to hemopericardium, and in rare circumstances may result in a false aneurysm of the LV.

Hemopericardium from rupture generally is a fatal event. The sites of rupture of the free wall have similar distribution in the anterior, posterior and lateral wall of the LV.

Usually, rupture of the free wall of the LV occurs three to five days after the onset of infarction, and there is a tear between the contracting and necrotic muscle.

Uncommonly, the rupture occurs at about the second week following the onset of infarction when there is removal of necrotic myocardium, and, in such cases, the rupture is through the center of the infarcted area.

Formation of False Aneurysm: This results from the rupture of the free wall, and the formation of a restricted pericardial hematoma. The patient survives.

With time, the periphery of the hematoma becomes organized to form the wall of the false aneurysm. The false aneurysm usually shows a relatively narrow communication with the cavity of the LV, and has a propensity to rupture.

These features are in contrast to that of true aneurysm, in which the communication with the left ventricular cavity is wide and there is a low tendency to rupture.

The ECG commonly shows persistent ST-T segmental elevation in those leads projecting toward the infarction.

The two-dimensional echocardiographic features of an LV false aneurysm are sudden discontinuity of the free wall of the LV and communication through a narrow neck into a saccular or globular cavity, which often contains a mural thrombus.

G. Rupture of the Heart

3. *Rupture of the Free Wall and False Aneurysm*

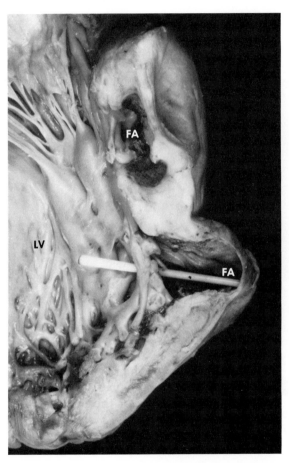

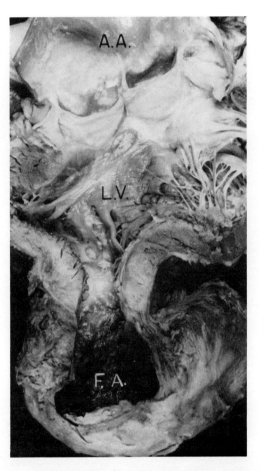

Fig. 69. Interior of the LV with section through the lateral wall of the LV, revealing two small false aneurysms. The lower one containing a probe is ruptured. Fig. 69 reproduced with permission of the American Heart Association Inc. From Vlodaver Z., Coe J. J., and Edwards J.E. Circulation 51:567, 1975a.

Fig. 70. Inside the LV showing a false aneurysm in the apical portion of the LV, with the classical feature of a narrow neck connecting with the LV cavity. Fig. 70 reproduced with permission from Gobel FL, Visudh Arom K, Edwards JE: Chest 59:23, 1971 FA: False aneurysm. AA: Ascending aorta

A. Contrast Two-Dimensional Echocardiography

Figures 73 and 74 visualize the heart structures following rapid injection of contrast material into a peripheral vein.

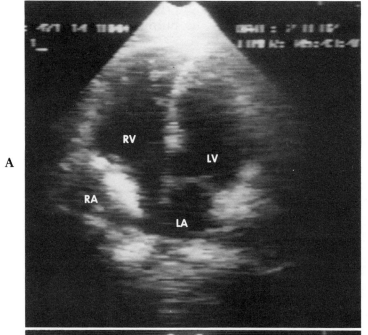

Fig. 73. Apical four-chamber view. **A,** Partial filling of the right atrium by contrast material following the injection into a peripheral vein.

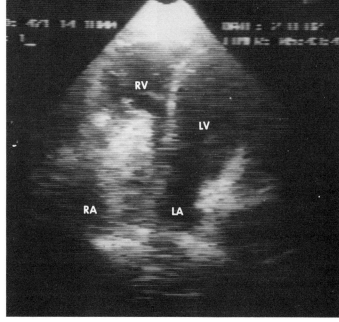

Fig. 73. B, Contrast material filling the right atrium and early transit into the right ventricle.

A. Contrast Two-Dimensional Echocardiography

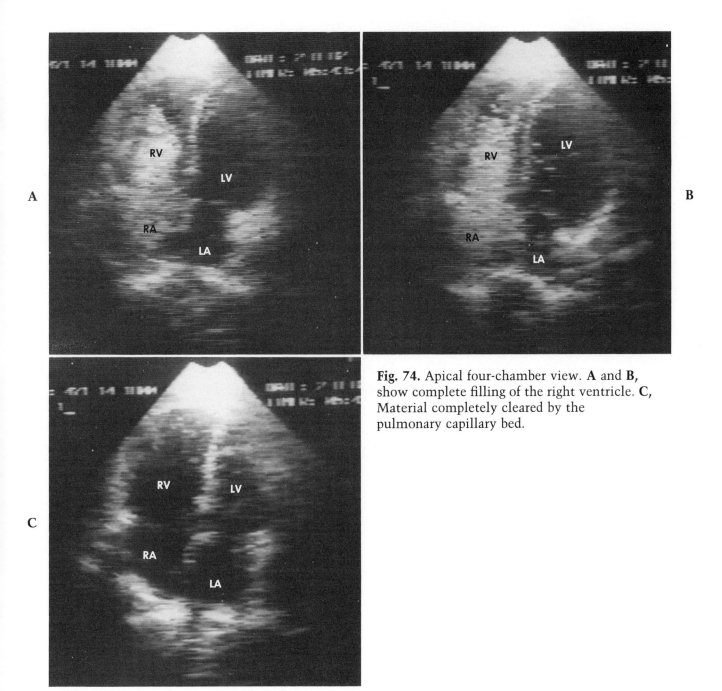

A

B

C

Fig. 74. Apical four-chamber view. **A** and **B,** show complete filling of the right ventricle. **C,** Material completely cleared by the pulmonary capillary bed.

B. Exercise Test Echocardiogram

Analysis of segmental wall motion abnormalities during and after physical stress can help detect coronary artery disease and may further predict its extent and severity.

Several forms of exercise have been used successfully with echocardiography to assess ventricular function during stress, specifically supine bicycle exercise, upright bicycle exercise, handgrip exercise and treadmill exercise. Echocardiographic tracings are recorded before and immediately after exercise.

Handgrip exercise: Echocardiography with handgrip exercise preceded echocardiography during dynamic exercise by a number of years because of the potential of obtaining optimal recordings during submaximal handgrip. Handgrip exercise produces little change in the diastolic dimension of the LV, increases the systolic dimension of the LV in normal subjects, but produces a reduction in the LV function in patients with ischemic heart disease.

However, the increases in heart rate and blood pressure products and in the myocardial oxygen requirements caused by handgrip exercise are not as large as the increase caused by dynamic exercise performed on a bicycle ergometer or on a treadmill.

Supine bicycle exercise: The use of echocardiography during supine dynamic exercise provides continuous real time images of the LV structures, demonstrates changes in the cardiac output and identifies wall motion abnormalities in patients with ischemic heart disease. Adjust the position of the subject, as positioning the patient at an angle between the supine and left lateral position sometimes results in more optimal recordings.

Treadmill exercise: Two-dimensional echocardiography performed immediately after treadmill exercise is a feasible technique in the assessment of ventricular wall motion abnormalities.

B. Exercise Test Echocardiogram

M-mode echocardiographic studies during and immediately after exercise testing have been of limited value because the M-mode study, unlike two-dimensional echocardiography, lacks spatial orientation and does not provide simultaneous visualization of adjacent structures.

Two-dimensional echocardiography immediately, 30 and 60 seconds after treadmill stress testing (which permits more vigorous exercise and greater oxygen consumption), is more likely than bicycle exercise and handgrip exercise to induce myocardial ischemia and therefore recognition of abnormal wall motion.

Its use in patients with prior myocardial infarction and abnormal wall motion at rest, may demonstrate new abnormalities in previously normal LV segments, or worsening of asynergia after exercise.

Lack of exercise-induced regional wall motion abnormalities does not exclude coronary artery disease.

B. Exercise Test Echocardiogram

LV echocardiogram from the patient shown on page 113, immediately after exercise treadmill test.

A

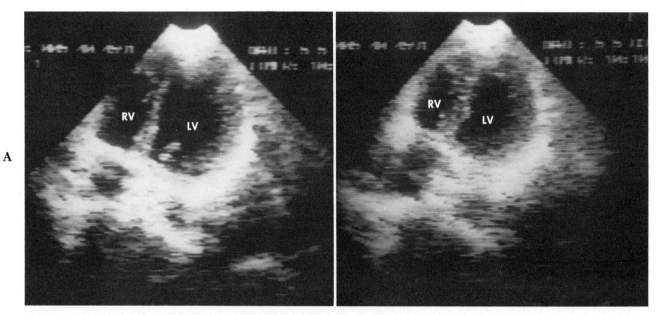

B

Fig. 77. Apical two-chamber view, with special inclination of the transducer for visualization of the inferior wall. **A,** Diastole and **B,** Systole, shows reduced systolic thickening of the inferoseptal segment of the LV.

C. Identification of Left Main Coronary Arterial Obstruction

The diagnosis of left main coronary artery disease is important in the management of patients with ischemic heart disease.

The apical cross-sectional approach and short axis view permits visualization of the left main coronary artery and its bifurcation and has the potential for detecting a left main coronary obstruction lesion.

Echocardiography is not routinely used because visualization of the left main coronary artery is possible in only 60% of cases even using multiple still-frame images. At present, coronary arteriographic findings are more predictable and convincing.

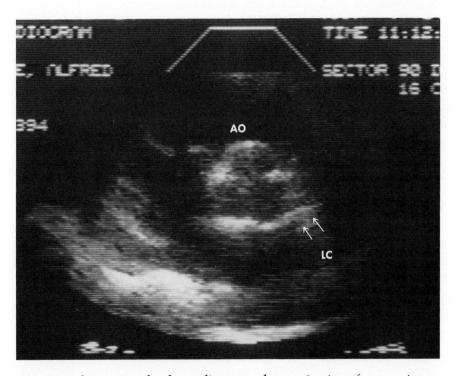

Fig. 78. Two-dimensional echocardiogram, short axis view, from patient with healed subendocardial inferior wall infarction, showing the main left coronary artery (LC) take off from the left coronary sinus (arrows). Bright echoes delineating the coronary arterial wall, representing calcified changes in the wall. No evidence of stenotic lesion.

D. Thrombolytic Therapy in Acute Myocardial Infarction

During the last decade efforts have been made and a variety of interventions designed to reduce the size of the infarction by decreasing oxygen demand or increasing supply. These have been validated in animal models and currently are the subject of clinical investigation.

In contrast to methods which reduce oxygen demand, early reperfusion may represent the most effective approach to limit myocardial necrosis.

Recently new methods have been introduced for non-surgical recanalization of coronary occlusion in patients with acute myocardial infarction utilizing selective intracoronary infusion or intravenous infusion of streptokinase. These methods are promising in the approach to re-establish the patency of coronary occlusion and achieve reperfusion in patients with acute myocardial infarction.

A relationship between coronary thrombosis and myocardial infarction has been known for many years, but the role of formation of thrombi in the pathogenesis of infarction has been controversial since pathologic studies have reported varying incidences of coronary thrombi at postmortem examination. Recent studies using coronary arteriography and clinical experience with emergency coronary bypass surgery have demonstrated that there is a high incidence of coronary occlusion by thrombus in patients with acute infarction.

Whether or not thrombosis is a primary or secondary factor in the pathogenesis of the infarction, it appears to have an important role in the extension of the process of ischemic injury once occlusion has occurred.

Thrombolytic agents produce activation of the fibrinolytic system which counters the coagulation.

A number of studies have been performed using streptokinase, urokinase and thrombolysin (a mixture of streptokinase and human plasmin).

D. Thrombolytic Therapy in Acute Myocardial Infarction

Streptokinase, the most widely used thrombolytic agent, is a non-enzymatic protein of hemolytic streptococci which produces indirect activation of fibrinolysis by the formation of an activator complex with plasminogen. This activator converts additional plasminogen to plasmin, the active protease which degrades fibrin to soluble complexes and results in the dissolution of the fibrin thrombus.

Intracoronary thrombolysis can be accomplished using similar procedures of coronary arteriography. The ideal patients for intracoronary thrombolysis are those presenting within the first few hours of symptoms of infarction and having ECG evidence of evolving acute infarction and who have no contraindication to anticoagulation. To achieve substantial salvage and prevent the evolution of necrosis, streptokinase infusion should be started within 3 to 4 hours of onset of the infarction.

An initial dose of streptokinase bolus of 10,000-25,000 units is often given, followed by continuous infusion (2,000-4,000 units per minute).

The total dosage of streptokinase is usually in the range of 200,000-400,000 units, and the average infusion duration is approximately 60-90 minutes.

The limitation in the application of this technique is the requirement of expensive technology and catheterization teams.

Intravenous administration of thrombolytic agents could be used in most community hospitals. It has the advantage over intracoronary infusion in that therapy can be started sooner after the onset of symptoms of acute infarction.

The total dosage of intravenous streptokinase is in the range of 1 million to 1-1/2 million units in 50 cc normal saline to be infused over 60 minutes.

Significant bleeding occurs in 5 to 7% of patients following streptokinase infusion.

D. Thrombolytic Therapy in Acute Myocardial Infarction

The methodology is currently not standardized. The quantitative assessment of the extent of myocardial salvage is not available and further evaluation of long term effects is needed.

Echocardiographic studies before and after thrombolytic therapy are important to determine the beneficial effects of reperfusion on left ventricular function. Electrocardiographic and enzyme indices, used to assess infarct size in experimental models and in patients, are probably not applicable to reperfusion.

Beneficial effects of reperfusion on left ventricular function have been suggested by improvement in the ejection fraction following thrombolysis.

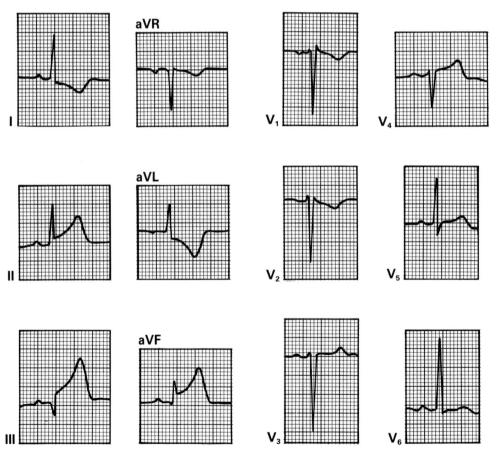

Fig. 79. A, ECG tracing from a patient with acute infarction, one hour after onset of symptoms, showing ST segment elevation on leads L2, L3, aVF, Q wave in L3, and inverted T waves in L1, aVL, V1 and V2 compatible with evolving inferior wall infarction.

D. Thrombolytic Therapy in Acute Myocardial Infarction

The ideal patients for thrombolytic therapy are patients presenting within the first few hours of symptoms of infarction.

Shown on this and the previous page are illustrations from a patient with classical symptoms of acute infarction and electrocardiographic evidence of acute evolving inferior wall infarction. Intravenous strep-tokinase was administered two hours after the onset of symptoms. Following the injection, there was normalization of ST segment elevation and relief of chest pain. The echocardiogram obtained the next day revealed adequate motion of the inferior wall, with only moderate reduced systolic thickening of the inferobasal segment of the LV, and normal function values, as seen with focal subendocardial infarction.

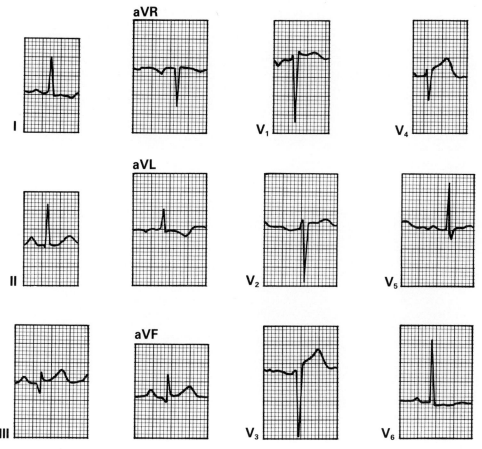

Fig. 79. B, ECG two hours following intravenous injection associated with relief of residual ischemic chest pain and with normalization of ST segment elevation, suggesting interruption of the ischemia. Small Q waves developed in leads L3 and aVF.

D. Thrombolytic Therapy in Acute Myocardial Infarction

LV echocardiogram from the patient illustrated on page 119 recorded 24 hours following the intravenous injection of streptokinase.

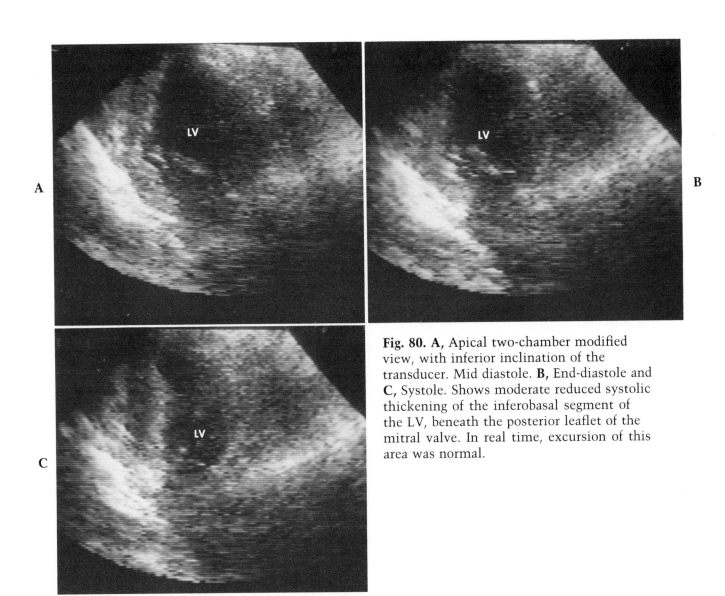

Fig. 80. A, Apical two-chamber modified view, with inferior inclination of the transducer. Mid diastole. **B,** End-diastole and **C,** Systole. Shows moderate reduced systolic thickening of the inferobasal segment of the LV, beneath the posterior leaflet of the mitral valve. In real time, excursion of this area was normal.

D. Thrombolytic Therapy in Acute Myocardial Infarction

Shown on this and the next page are illustrations from a patient with acute anteroseptal infarction, in whom intravenous injection of streptokinase was associated with relief of chest pain and normalization of ST segment elevation. This was administered four hours after the onset of symptoms. The next day the echocardiogram revealed hypokinesis and reduced systolic thickening of the apical segment of the LV; the LV function values were moderately reduced.

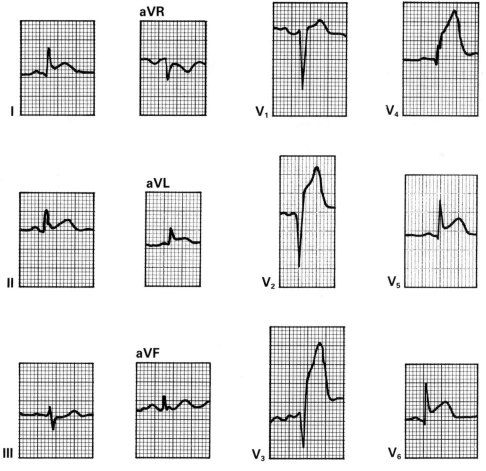

Fig. 81. A, ECG tracing from a patient admitted for severe chest pain, showing ST elevation and Q waves in precordal leads consistent with acute evolving anteroseptal infarction.

D. Thrombolytic Therapy in Acute Myocardial Infarction

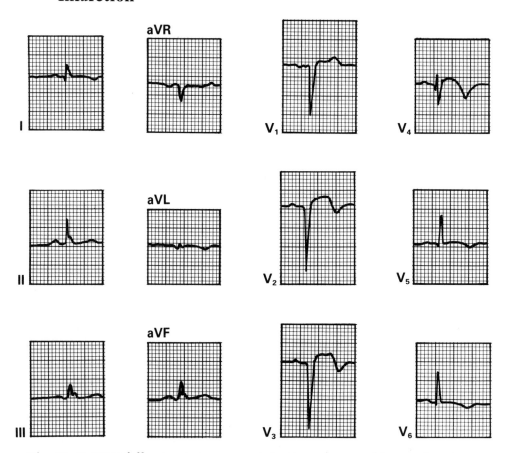

Fig. 81. B, ECG following intravenous injection of streptokinase, showing normalization of ST segment elevation, suggesting interruption of ischemia, but persistence of Q waves, of the infarcted tissue.

D. Thrombolytic Therapy in Acute Myocardial Infarction

LV echocardiogram from the patient shown on page 121 with acute anteroseptal infarction recorded 24 hours after intravenous injection of streptokinase.

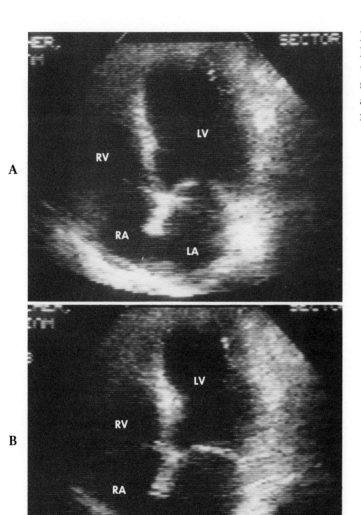

Fig. 82. Apical four-chamber views. **A,** Diastole. **B,** Systole, showing reduced systolic thickening and hypokinesis of the distal segment of the interventricular septum and apical portion of the LV. LV function moderate reduced: ejection fraction 50%.

ECHOCARDIOGRAM PROFILES FOR THE CARDIAC REHABILITATION PROGRAM

LV FUNCTION

LV ECHO	I NORMAL	II ABNORMAL MODERATE	III POOR
E. FRACTION	≥60	59-50	≤49
MEAN VCF	≥1.00	0.99-0.70	≤0.69
% Δ SEPTUM	≥30	29-15	≤14
% Δ INFERIOR WALL	≥45	44-30	≤29
MOTION SEPTUM	≥5 mm	HYPOKINESIS 4-3 mm	AKINESIS 1-0 mm
MOTION INFERIOR	≥8 mm	HYPOKINESIS 7-5 mm	AKINESIS 2-0 mm

A. Introduction

The concept of cardiac rehabilitation is that patients with acute or chronic ischemic heart disease can and should return to normal living.

Cardiac rehabilitation includes medical care, prescribed and regular physical activity, diagnosis with emphasis in assessment of patient's physical, emotional, educational and vocational function status, and prevention of risk factors. Cardiac rehabilitation provides medical and nursing services, education for the patient and his family, occupational therapy, exercise leaders, dietitian, sexual education, social services, psychology support and stress management. All these services are integrated into one team, the cardiac team.

The responsibility to restore the patient with acute infarction to independence and productive living rests in the primary physician, working closely with the cardiac team.

The cardiac team approaches the patient as soon as he is stabilized in the coronary care unit and follows and works with the patient's family through his hospitalization, convalescence and complete recovery.

After myocardial infarction, there are three phases in cardiac rehabilitation.

B. Phase I—Inpatient Program

This is related to the acute care in the coronary care unit and in the post-coronary care area and begins when the patient is declared electrically and hemodynamically stable.

Benefits of early ambulation and the inpatient cardiac rehabilitation program include: prevention of deconditioning, a decrease in thromboembolic complications, reduction in patient's anxiety and depression.

Early in the Inpatient Program regular exercise activities of a very low level are prescribed by the primary physician and followed with electrocardiographic monitoring.

Early and regular exercise activities can reassure the patient of his ability to perform activities safely, and can decrease his anxiety and that of his spouse.

The goals of physical exercise in the Inpatient Program are the improvement and maintenance of habitual neuromuscular relaxation, efficient breathing to prevent hyperventilation and promotion of venous circulation to prevent thromboembolic complications.

The exercises are performed twice a day while the patient continues to be monitored by telemetric electrocardiography to detect arrhythmias or ischemic changes.

B. Phase I—Inpatient Program

In the Coronary Care or Intensive Care Units for post coronary bypass patients, in an average stay of 3 to 5 days, patients undergo a progressive active/passive range of motion exercises, going from 5 to 20 minutes a day, several times a day, as well as self-care in the use of a bedside commode. Physical activity is carried out under cardiac monitoring and serious signs of excessive myocardial work such as chest pain, marked dyspnea, or a heart rate greater than 120 at this early stage, indicates a need to reduce the rate of physical activity.

At this phase, the resting heart rate should be about 20 beats above resting level for post myocardial infarction patients and 30 beats for post coronary bypass surgery patients. A drop in blood pressure, significant serious arrhythmias or ST-T segment depression on ECG monitoring during the exercise indicates that the exercise should be discontinued. With normalization of blood pressure and heart rhythm and stabilization of ST-T segment, exercise activities can be reinstated.

During the remainder of the hospital stay (average of 10 to 14 days), and in the absence of cardiac complications, the levels of physical activity may be progressively increased to approximately what the patient will be doing at home, usually to a level of 3 to 4 METS. Physical activity consists primarily of self-care and walking, which at first, can be performed in the room, then in the corridor, or can be done on a bicycle ergometer. The duration of walking is increased gradually to 20 to 30 minutes several times a day.

Heart rate and blood pressure are checked before and at the peak of exercise for inappropriate elevations or insufficient blood pressure response to exercise.

The occupational therapist instructs the patient in the principles and techniques of energy conservation that will make it possible for the patient to live in greater freedom, independence, and safety during the convalescent and recovery phases.

D. LV Echocardiographic Patterns; Phase I—Inhospital Program

Echocardiography in patients participating in a cardiac rehabilitation program after acute myocardial infarction is an important screening procedure for identifying patients with limited exercise tolerance to other illness that might be associated with myocardial infarction, as patients with large pericardial effusion, valvular disease, cardiomyopathy.

D. LV Echocardiographic Patterns; Phase I—Inhospital Program

The patients were divided into three groups on the basis of M-mode echocardiographic motion and contraction patterns of the LV wall and LV function values (See figures 83 and 84)

LV ECHO PATTERNS

GROUP	MOTION INFARCTED WALL	SYSTOLIC THICKENING INFARCTED WALL	LV FUNCTION
I 25	NORMAL	NORMAL	NORMAL
II 31	HYPOKINESIS	± ↓	± ↓
III 11	AKINESIS	↓	↓

Fig. 83. Table M-mode LV echocardiogram motion and contraction patterns. Fig. 83 used with permission of The C. V. Mosby Company from Vlodaver Z., Boyum A., Gesundheit S., Long S., Peterson R., Spenny E., Thorsen R. D. Heart and Lung, 12:351, 1983.

Group I: Patients with normal motion and contraction patterns of the LV wall and normal LV function.

Group II: Patients with hypokinesis (reduced motion) either of the IV septum or the inferior wall and moderately reduced LV function values.

Group III: Patients with akinesis (almost no motion) and poor contraction patterns of the IV septum or inferior wall, and markedly reduced LV function values.

D. LV Echocardiographic Patterns; Phase I—Inhospital Program

LV FUNCTION

LV ECHO	I NORMAL	II ABNORMAL MODERATE	III POOR
E. FRACTION	≥60	59-50	≤49
MEAN VCF	≥1.00	0.99-0.70	≤0.69
% Δ SEPTUM	≥30	29-15	≤14
% Δ INFERIOR WALL	≥45	44-30	≤29
MOTION SEPTUM	≥5 mm	HYPOKINESIS 4-3 mm	AKINESIS 1-0 mm
MOTION INFERIOR	≥8 mm	HYPOKINESIS 7-5 mm	AKINESIS 2-0 mm

Fig. 84. Table M-mode LV echocardiographic function values. Fig. 84 used with permission of The C. V. Mosby Company from Vlodaver Z., Boyum A., Gesundheit S., Long S., Peterson R., Spenny E., Thorsen R. D. Heart and Lung, 12:351, 1983.

D. LV Echocardiographic Patterns; Phase I—Inhospital Program

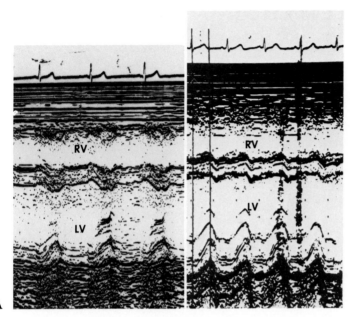

A   B

Fig. 85. M-mode LV echocardiograms from patients with acute myocardial infarction. **A,** From a patient in group I with subendocardial infarction of the inferior wall showing normal motion of the IV septum and inferior wall, but reduced systolic thickening of inferior wall. LV function values are within normal limits. EF: 64%. **B,** From a patient in group II, with acute anteroseptal subendocardial infarction, showing hypokinesis and reduced systolic thickening of the IV septum. LV function values are moderately reduced. EF: 55%. Fig. 85 used with permission by The C. V. Mosby Company from Vlodaver Z., Boyum A., Gesundheit S., Long S., Peterson R., Spenny E., Thorsen R. D. Heart and Lung, 12:351, 1983.

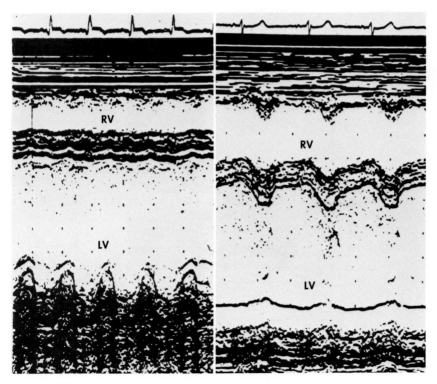

A   B

Fig. 86. M-mode LV echocardiograms from patients in group III. **A,** From a patient with acute anterior wall infarction. The LV is enlarged. There is akinesis and poor systolic thickening of the IV septum. LV function is reduced. EF: 45%; mean VCF: 0.78cm/sec; thickening of the septum: 9%. **B,** From a patient with acute extensive inferior wall infarction, showing enlarged LV, akinesis of the inferior wall, and hyperkinetic IV septum. EF: 46%; mean VCF: 0.72cm/sec; thickening of the inferior wall: 10%.

SECTION VI

PHASE II—OUTPATIENT CARDIAC EXERCISE PROGRAM

ALLAN BOYUM, M.D.
SIM GESUNDHEIT, M.D.
STEVEN LONG, M.D.
ROBERT PETERSON, M.D.
EDWARD A. SPENNY, M.D.
R. DOUGLAS THORSEN, M.D.
ZEEV VLODAVER, M.D.

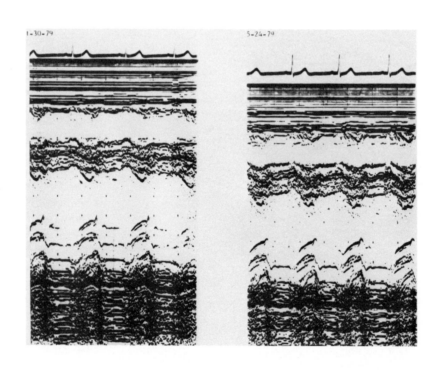

A. Introduction

Phase II begins 1 to 2 weeks after patient dismissal from the hospital and continues for three months. Within this time the myocardial scar will have developed and the patient will have safely reached the exercise tolerance which permits his return to work.

During this phase and after recovery, an individually planned, progressively increasing physical activity program is prescribed, based on the telemetric electrocardiographic monitoring during exercise, a submaximal exercise stress test and a noninvasive evaluation of the LV function.

Regular exercise and physical activity may produce an increasing feeling of physical well-being and assists in providing the patient with self assertiveness and psychological drive.

The submaximal endurance training results in a decrease of the resting heart rate, decrease in the systolic and diastolic blood pressure, and a decrease of heart rate and blood pressure in response to specific levels of submaximal work load, which constitute an increase in efficiency of myocardial work.

Also it is well documented that cardiac output, stroke volume and end diastolic volume all tend to increase with submaximal training.

An exercise prescription should define the intensity, the duration and the frequency of the individual regular exercise.

Walking, bicycling, swimming and calisthenics, at least 30 minutes and three times a week, are desirable types of endurance exercise.

The intensity of the exercise should not exceed 70% of the maximal, age-related, predicted heart rate, or the heart rate at which cardiac symptoms or signs appeared during the stress test.

Isometric exercise should be avoided, because of the associated effect on blood pressure.

A. Introduction

The use of electrocardiographic telemetry dynamic monitoring during exercise training is beneficial for early detection of significant ventricular arrhythmias, ischemic changes, and for assessing exercise training effects on patients following acute myocardial infarction. A study of 50 patients in the three month Outpatient Exercise Program revealed 18% of the patients developed serious ventricular arrhythmias during the program.

With appropriate antiarrhythmic medications, the incidence was reduced to 3% by the end of the program.

Ischemic changes (ST-T changes) during exercise were observed in 22% of the outpatients. 74% of these had atypical or no symptoms. 50% of the patients with serious arrhythmias responded to modified exercise prescriptions and/or therapeutical adjustments.

B. Clinical Evaluation

Seventy-five patients with acute myocardial infarction, who participated in an Inpatient Cardiac Rehabilitation Program, were followed for three months in an Outpatient Program.

Eight patients in this group developed ECG findings of new infarction after coronary bypass surgery.

All patients exercised daily during the inpatient program, and every other day as outpatients. Exercise activities were monitored with ECG telemetry, which recorded heart rate and ST-T segment changes. Blood pressure was recorded before and at peak of exercise.

M-mode echocardiogram studies were performed on each patient one week and three months after acute infarction.

The patients were classified into four groups on the basis of echocardiographic motion and systolic thickening of the LV wall and their LV function values.

Group I consisted of 25 patients with normal motion and contraction pattern of the LV wall and normal LV function values. Group II included 31 patients with hypokinesis of either the IV septum or the inferior wall, and moderately reduced LV function values. Group III was 11 patients with akinesis and poor systolic thickening of the infarcted area, and Group IV was composed of 8 patients after coronary bypass surgery with new Q waves in the electrocardiogram and dyskinesis of the IV septum, or inferior wall, and relatively normal or mildly reduced LV function values.

This study showed that abnormalities in the motion and contraction pattern of the LV wall corresponded to the ECG site of infarction in most cases of anteroseptal and/or inferior wall infarction. No correlation was found in cases of lateral infarction.

B. Clinical Evaluation

Patients with normal LV function after acute MI probably have nonextensive or subendocardial infarction. Each of these cases was restudied with two-dimensional echocardiography to confirm the M-mode findings. LV echo findings and the information obtained from continuous ECG monitoring during exercise activities were of important practical application in the determination of the prognosis of these patients.

Most patients in Groups I and IV, with normal LV function values, had a LV chamber of normal size, a lower incidence of serious ventricular arrhythmias during the acute stages of their infarction, and fewer ischemic changes during the three months followup.

In Group II, patients with moderately reduced LV function, 29% showed an enlarged LV, 64% showed serious arrhythmias in the acute stage of the infarction, and 10% showed ischemic changes. Group III, patients with poor LV function and akinesis of the infarcted area, showed higher incidence of LV enlargement (45%), serious arrhythmias (54%) and ischemic changes (55%) in the three months followup. Myocardial infarction in this group of patients was probably very extensive.

LV hypertrophy was present in 56% of the patients and was a common finding in ischemic heart disease, probably related to systemic hypertension in these patients.

Improvement of LV function occurred in 77% of the patients participating in the three month Outpatient Program, and was associated with improvement in their exercise tolerance.

B. Clinical Evaluation

LV function values improved in almost all the patients in Group I, and in two thirds of the patients of Groups II and III by the end of the three month Outpatient Exercise Program.

In 17 patients with deteriorated or poor LV function three months after infarction, there was an associated LV enlargement (57%), ischemic changes (29%), and/or reduced exercise tolerance (82%).

C. LV Echocardiogram Profiles

LV echocardiogram with normal pattern and improved LV function. M-mode echocardiographic findings were confirmed in all the cases with two-dimensional echocardiographic evaluation.

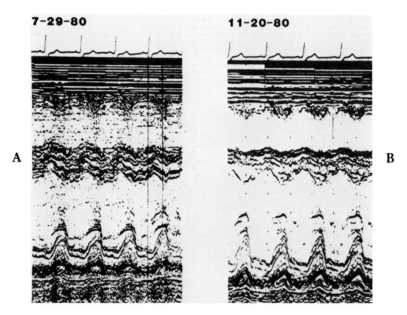

Fig. 87. M-mode LV echocardiogram from a patient in Group I, with acute anteroseptal subendocardial infarction. **A,** One week after admission shows normal motion of the IVS and PW, with reduced systolic thickening of the IVS. EF: 66%. **B,** Three months later, the LV echocardiogram pattern remained unchanged; the LV function values improved. EF: 80%. ECG monitoring during exercise showed sinus rhythm, regular; ST-T segment was stable; exercise tolerance (double product of heart rate and blood pressure) significantly improved.

B. Su

D
etiolo;
apists
factor
delay

(
in the
six m
year.

T
traini
capac
partic
patin;

ercise
100 p
patie
("nor
them
show

C. LV Echocardiogram Profiles

LV echocardiogram with improved LV motion pattern and function values. Shown on this page are illustrations from a patient in group II, with acute inferior wall infarction and moderately reduced LV function values, and significant improvement in the LV echocardiographic pattern, three months later.

ECG monitoring during exercise, revealed sinus rhythm, regular; ST-T segment stable, exercise tolerance improved; level of activity of 5 METS.

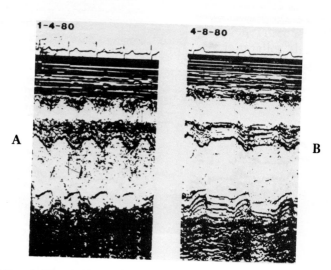

Fig. 88. A, LV echocardiogram one week after admission, showing hypokinesis and reduced systolic thickening of the PW. EF: 54%. **B,** Three months later, showing improvement in the motion and systolic thickening of the PW. EF: 66%. Fig. 88 used with permission of The C. V. Mosby Company from Vlodaver Z., Boyum A., Gesundheit S., Long S., Peterson R., Spenny E., Thorsen R. D. Heart and Lung, 12:351, 1983.

B. Survey

1. *Risk Factors:*

Family History of Myocardial Infarction: (Relatives died of a heart attack before the age of 60.) Figure 95 shows that 56% of the patients' mothers or fathers died of heart attack before the age of 60.

Family History of Hypertension, Hyperlipidemia, Diabetes: Figure 96. 48% of their parents or siblings had hypertension, 27% diabetes and 17% hyperlipidemia.

Smoking: 82% of the patients were cigarette smokers before their heart attack. Two thirds of the patients quit smoking after their heart attack.

Our findings are comparable with other epidemiological studies showing that individuals with these risk factors are more likely to develop ischemic heart disease.

B. Survey

1. *Risk Factors:*

FAMILY HISTORY OF MYOCARDIAL INFARCTION
(Relatives Died of Heart Attack Before the Age of 60)

Mother or Father	Siblings	Other Relatives
56	16	46

Fig. 95.

FAMILY HISTORY OF PARENTS AND SIBLINGS

High Blood Pressure	High Cholesterol, Triglycerides or Other Blood Lipids	Diabetes	Heart Surgery	Congenital Heart Disease
48	17	27	14	9

Fig. 96.

B. Survey

2. *Diet:*

During their hospitalization with acute myocardial infarction, the patients received a standard coronary diet low in cholesterol, no added salt and no caffeine.

These restrictions may also have included a calorie restriction for diabetes or obesity.

The patients' nutritional and educational needs were assessed by the dietitian. Diet instructions were provided according to the assessment. This survey, one year after their heart attack, indicated that both participants and non-participants in the exercise program were able to decrease cholesterol and sodium intake.

Most of the patients were avoiding caffeine (changed to decaffeinated coffee), consuming 0 to 3 eggs per week, using margarine, cooking with little salt, limiting fat intake and reading food labels.

Diet adherence to a calorie-controlled diet was a problem for all overweight patients. Figure 97: Weight gain was a significant problem for non-participants in the program, and may be related to a lack of regular exercise.

For participants at the time of the survey, 49% of the group were overweight, an increase of 4% since their participation in the inpatient program. For non-participants at the time of the survey, 76% of the group were overweight, an increase of 20%.

B. Survey

2. *Diet:*

DIET AND WEIGHT STATUS
OVERWEIGHT POPULATION

	66 PARTICIPANTS		34 NONPARTICIPANTS	
	INPATIENTS	SURVEY	INPATIENTS	SURVEY
OVERWEIGHT— NON CALORIE CONTROL DIET	8	21	6	19
	12%	32%	18%	56%
OVERWEIGHT— CALORIE CONTROL DIET	22	11	13	7
	33%	17%	38%	20%
TOTAL	30	32	19	26
	45%	49%	56%	76%

Fig. 97

B. Survey

3. *Occupation:*

More coronary patients now return to work than was the case two decades ago. The criteria for a successful rehabilitation program after myocardial infarction involves return to gainful employment or to independent living. This will lead to a reduction of the economic burden of the myocardial infarction on the patient's family and his community, through a decrease in the need for convalescent care, and an increase in the number who return to work.

Most of the patients (89%) were employed before their heart attack. The number of patients retired or not working increased from 11% before their heart attack to 30% after their heart attack. This increase was more significant in the non-participant group in the cardiac rehabilitation program.

Figure 98, the number of patients on medical disability was larger among the non-participants (participants 7.6%; non-participants 23.5%). 16.6% of the participants in the exercise program took different jobs after their heart attack, compared to 2.9% of non-participants.

These figures might indicate that those following a rehabilitation exercise program are likely to be physically more able to return to work than cardiac patients who do not.

It may also indicate that participants are more educated and understand their physical limitations, thus they are more willing to make vocational changes.

The rehabilitation process develops self-confidence and independence making it easier for the participants to resume an active role, even if they have to take a different job.

B. Survey

3. *Occupation:*

MEDICAL DISABILITY AFTER HEART ATTACK

	YES	NO	NO INFORMATION
PARTICIPANTS 66	5	60	1
	7.6%	90.9%	1.5%
NONPARTICIPANTS 34	8	26	0
	23.5%	76.5%	0%
TOTAL 100	13	86	1

Fig. 98

B. Survey

4. *Exercise and Physical Activities*

Most of the patients started their regular exercise activities after they experienced their heart attack.

Only 13% of these patients were exercising before their heart attack. The one year followup survey revealed that 63.6% of the participants continued with moderate to active exercise, compared to 41% of nonparticipants (figure 99). The participants in a regular exercise program are able to achieve a higher level of submaximal exercise, compared to non-participants, and are more free of symptoms during their exercise activities (figure 100, MET Level; figure 101, Chest Pain, Shortness of Breath with Moderate Exercise).

B. Survey

4. *Exercise and Physical Activities*

**PHYSICAL ACTIVITY
REGULAR EXERCISE**

	NO	VERY LITTLE TO LITTLE	MODERATE	ACTIVE TO VERY ACTIVE
PARTICIPANTS 66	21	3	22	20
	31.8%	4.5%	33.3%	30.3%
NONPARTICIPANTS 34	17	3	6	8
	50%	8.8%	17.6%	23.4%
TOTAL 100	38	6	28	28

Fig. 99

B. Survey

4. *Exercise and Physical Activities*

MET LEVEL
MONITORED SUBMAXIMAL EXERCISE SESSION

	NO INFORMATION	2-3 METS	3.1-4.0 METS	≥4.1 METS
PARTICIPANTS 66	1	14	37	14
	1.5%	21.2%	56.1%	21.2%
NONPARTICIPANTS 34	1	16	14	3
	2.9%	47.1%	41.2%	8.8%
TOTAL 100	2	30	51	17

Fig. 100

B. Survey

4. *Exercise and Physical Activities*

QUESTION: Experience Discomfort, Chest Pain, or Shortness of Breath with Moderate Exercise?

	NO ANSWER	NO SYMPTOMS	SHORTNESS OF BREATH	ANGINA	SHORTNESS OF BREATH + ANGINA	OTHER DISCOMFORT
PARTICIPANTS 66	2	55	6	1	1	1
	3.0%	83.3%	9.1%	1.5% 12.1%	1.5%	1.5%
NONPARTICIPANTS 34	5	15	5	2	3	4
	14.7%	44.1%	14.7%	5.9% 29.4%	8.8%	11.8%
TOTAL 100	7	70	11	3	4	5

RAW CHI SQUARE: 0.0019
CRAMER'S V: 0.43682

Fig. 101

C. LV Echocardiographic Profiles

Shown on this and the next page are LV echocardiograms from a 46 year old man with a history of angina and hypertension for several years, prior to myocardial infarction.

The LV function was significantly reduced following acute infarction of the inferior wall.

The study was repeated three months and a half year following his heart attack. The study shows improvement in the motion and systolic thickening of the posterior wall. During this period of time, the patient was active in a regular supervised exercise program; his LV function and exercise tolerance were improved.

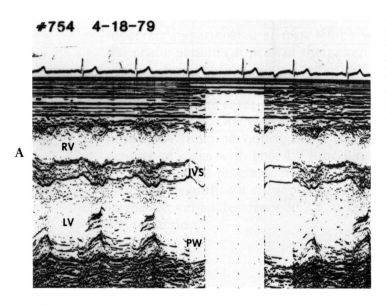

Fig. 103. M-mode LV echocardiogram, eight months prior to myocardial infarction, showing normal size of the LV (D:50mm), mild hypertrophy of the LV wall. EF: 71%; thickening of the septum: 42%; thickening of the PW: 83%. Normal motion and systolic thickening of the IVS and posterior wall.

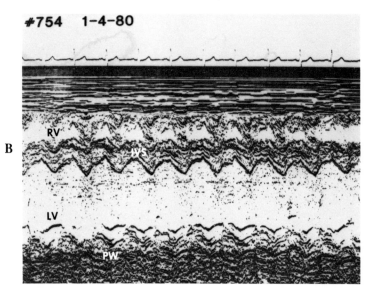

Fig. 104. M-mode LV echocardiogram, three days after the heart attack showing hypokinesis and reduced systolic thickening of the posterior wall. The motion of the IVS is relatively hyperkinetic. The LV function has deteriorated. EF: 43%; thickening of the IVS: 44%; thickening of the PW: 40%.

C. LV Echocardiographic Profiles

M-mode LV echocardiographic recordings from the patient illustrated on page 162 following myocardial infarction. The patient participated in a three month outpatient cardiac rehabilitation program, and, since then, in a regular conditioning exercise program. His level of activity is equivalent to 7 METS.

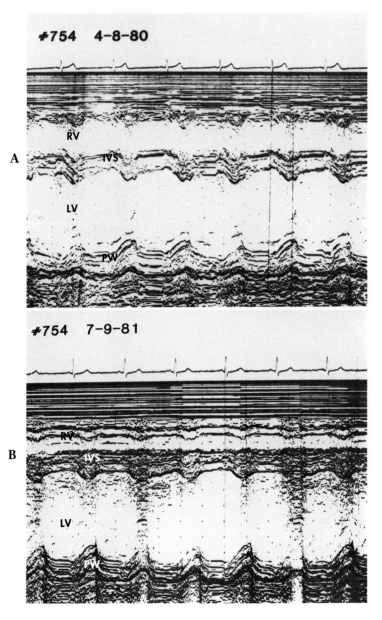

Fig. 105. A, M-mode LV echocardiogram three months after the myocardial infarction, showing improvement in the motion and systolic thickening of the posterior wall. LV function values are improved to the lower range of normal: EF: 63%; thickening of the PW: 76%.

Fig. 105. B, M-mode study one and a half years post infarction. The motion pattern of the LV wall and LV function remain unchanged. EF: 63%.

C. LV Echocardiographic Profiles

Shown on this page are illustrations of a patient with previous acute inferior wall infarction, participating in a regular exercise program. His LV echocardiographic pattern and exercise tolerance have significantly improved.

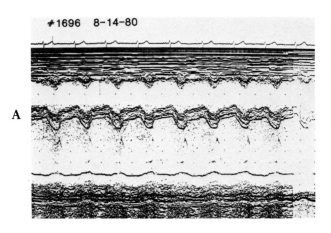

Fig. 106. A, LV echocardiogram 1 week following admission, showing akinesis and reduced systolic thickening of the PW, and relatively hyperkinetic IVS. LVD: 60 mm; EF: 52%; ET: 0.260 sec; mean VCF: 0.72cm/sec; thickening of the IVS:30%; PW:6; level of activity: 1 ½ METS.

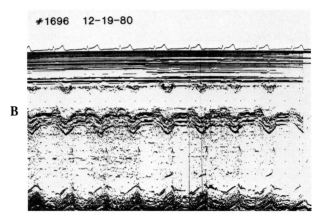

Fig. 106. B, Four months following the acute infarction, participant in the Outpatient Exercise Program. Asymptomatic during exercise. Level of activity: 4 METS; LVD:58mm; EF:56%; mean VCF:0.72cm/sec; thickening of the IVS: 30%; PW:15; motion of the PW improved.

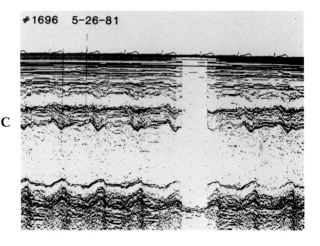

Fig. 106. C, Five months after patient participated in a regular exercise program. LVD reduced. LV function improved: EF: 60%; thickening of the PW:25%; level of activity: 6-7 METS. ECG monitoring during exercise showed sinus rhythm, regular. ST-T segment stable during activities.

C. LV Echocardiographic Profiles

Illustrations from a patient with acute anteroseptal infarction participating in a regular exercise program; his level of activity is 5 METS. In spite of his LV function being mildly reduced, the patient is free of symptoms during exercise activities, and his tolerance to moderately intensive exercise is good.

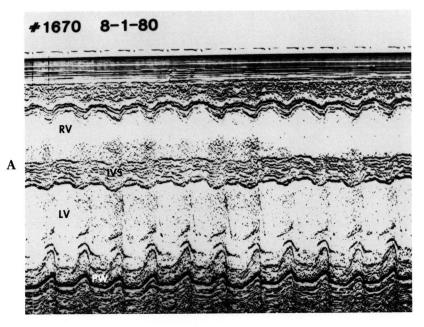

Fig. 107. A, M-mode LV echocardiogram 4 days after acute infarction of the anteroseptal wall, showing moderate hypokinesis and reduced systolic thickening of the IVS. LVD: 50mm; EF: 59%; moderately reduced.

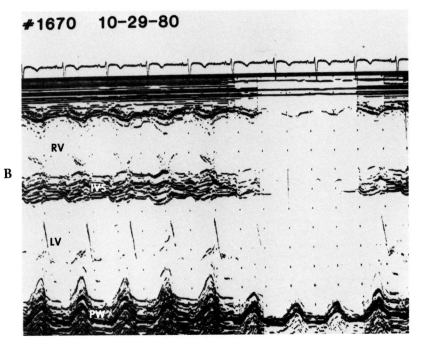

Fig. 107. B, Three months following the infarction. LV: 54mm; EF: 60%. Motion of the IVS remains hypokinetic.

C. LV Echocardiographic Profiles

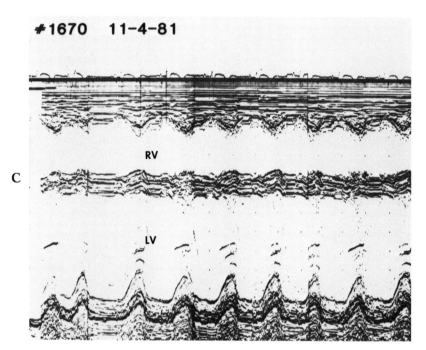

Fig. 107. C, Year later, M-mode study revealed hypokinesis and reduced systolic thickening of the IVS. LVD: 55mm; EF: 58%—the findings unchanged since previous study.

C. LV Echocardiographic Profiles

Shown on this page echocardiograms of a patient with previous coronary bypass surgery for angina pectoris. Two years later he developed acute myocardial infarction of the inferior wall. The patient participated in a three month outpatient exercise program and continued with regular exercise, without symptoms and with improvement in his exercise tolerance. Level of activities: 6 METS.

The motion and systolic thickening of the inferior wall appears improved two years after the myocardial infarction.

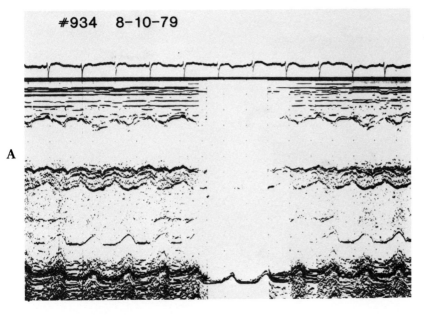

Fig. 108. A, LV echocardiogram three days following acute infarction, showing hypokinesis and reduced systolic thickening of the posterior wall. LVD: 52mm; EF: 58%; thickening of the PW: 38%.

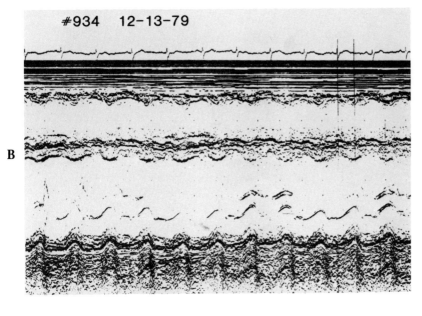

Fig. 108. B, Three months into the outpatient exercise program, patient is asymptomatic. Motion and systolic thickening of the inferior wall is unchanged since previous study. LVD: 53mm; EF: 58%; thickening of the PW: 38%.

C. Echocardiographic Profiles

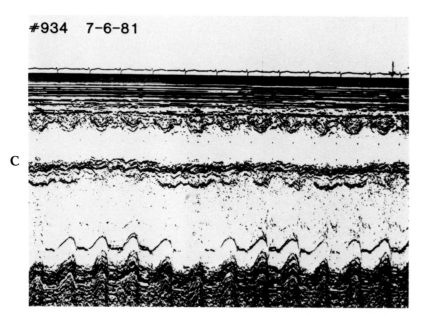

#934   7-6-81

C

Fig. 108. C, Study repeated 1½ years later, shows improved motion and systolic thickening of the inferior wall. LV function unchanged. EF: 60%; thickening of the PW: 57%.

C. LV Echocardiographic Profiles

Illustrations from a patient with acute inferolateral acute infarction, not participating in regular exercise program. Study repeated two years following his heart attack, revealed enlargement of the LV and deterioration in the LV function. Patient's exercise tolerance was poor.

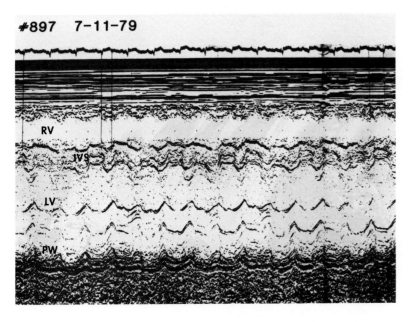

Fig. 109. M-mode LV echocardiogram, four days following acute inferolateral infarction showing hypokinesis and reduced systolic thickening of the PW. LVD: 60mm; LV EF: 60%.

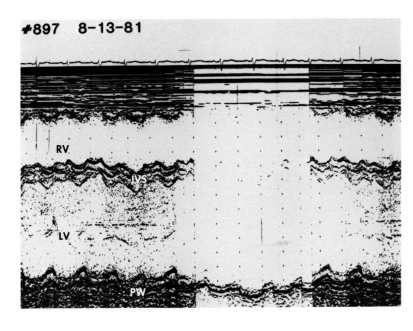

Fig. 110. Two years later, M-mode LV echocardiogram showing increased size of the LV and reduced LV function. LVD: 68mm; LV EF: 47%.

SURGICAL ASPECTS OF ACUTE MYOCARDIAL INFARCTION

PAUL G. GANNON, M.D.
EVAN F. LINDBERG, M.D.

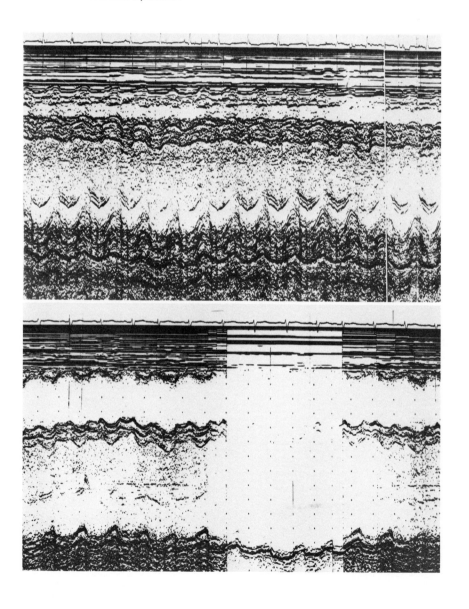

A. Introduction

Within the last five years there have been two significant developments in the treatment of acute myocardial infarction that have greatly influenced the outlook for survival of the patient and salvage of myocardium.

The most striking of these developments is the use of intracoronary or intravenous streptokinase for the dissolving of the clot in the coronary artery which accompanies acute myocardial infarction.

The other is the use of the percutaneous transluminal balloon arterioplasty technique for unblocking critically narrowed coronary arteries associated with symptoms of impending infarction.

The use of streptokinase for dissolving thrombosed arteries has been in practice for many years, but the application of this technique to the acutely thrombosed coronary artery is of more recent origin.

If the diagnosis of acute myocardial infarction is suspected, then 1.5 million units of streptokinase can be given intravenously with the expectation that approximately 70% of the acutely thrombosed arteries will open up. This can be confirmed by resolution of changes of acute myocardial infarction in the ECG.

Approximately 80% of the acutely occluded coronary arteries can have the thrombus lysed in where intracoronary streptokinase is injected by way of the coronary angiographic catheter. In this instance much less streptokinase is needed because of the concentration of the streptokinase into the occluded artery itself.

Because it is now appreciated that approximately 90% of all acute myocardial infarctions are associated with complete occlusion of the coronary artery feeding the affected musculature, it becomes much more important to treat the thrombosis aggressively if life and myocardium is to be preserved.

A. Introduction

For this reason the heart catheterization laboratory has evolved into a therapeutic tool rather than simply a diagnostic tool as has been the case in the past.

The next decade will witness a marked increase in the aggressive management of acute coronary thrombosis.

When the patient presents to the emergency room with physical findings and laboratory findings compatible with an acute coronary thrombosis, the patient can be directly transferred to the heart catheterization laboratory where emergency angiography can demonstrate the coronary anatomy and pathology. If only one vessel is occluded and the others are not seriously stenosed, then intracoronary streptokinase can be administered until lysis of the clot occurs. If there is a severe narrowing at the point of thrombosis demonstrated after lysis of the clot, this can be treated acutely with percutaneous balloon dilatation. Those patients who are successfully managed by these techniques can be discharged from the hospital after a few days. If the residual narrowing is not so severe as to demand balloon dilatation or bypass surgery, then the patient may be treated with long term anticoagulants alone.

If the patient has more than one coronary artery severely involved with the obstructing process, then the cardiologist has the option to lyse the clot with intracoronary streptokinase and then to transfer the patient to the operating room where definitive surgery can be performed, i.e. bypass to the recently thrombosed artery as well as to one or more severely obstructed coronaries.

A. Introduction

The postoperative convalescence following this approach can be shorter than the usual two week hospitalization following an acute myocardial infarction.

In the case where the heart catheterization laboratory is not immediately available, the patient can be treated with intravenous streptokinase and then can be transferred with less risk in an elective manner to the hospital having a heart catheterization lab. Then at an appropriate interval of a day or two, the patient can undergo coronary arteriography with determination of whether balloon dilatation or coronary bypass surgery or long term anticoagulation alone is indicated.

The second pathological fact that determines the effectiveness of aggressive management of acute myocardial infarction is the knowledge that the myocardium in the area involved with the coronary thrombosis is not irreversibly damaged at once. Rather the time factor is important in that the damage is progressive over an 8 hour period from the time of the occlusion of the coronary artery.

A. Introduction

Within the first hour or two, the changes are largely reversible, but beyond that time progressively more and more of the myocardium undergoes irreversible changes so that by 8 hours, generally the damage has been completed and acute revascularization via streptokinase or balloon dilatation or bypass surgery will not be effective in the myocardium.

B. Intervention for Acute Coronary Occlusion

1. *Thrombolytic Therapy with Streptokinase*

When the patient presents to the physician with evidence of acute myocardial infarction, the conventional treatment is to confine the patient to the coronary care unit where ECG monitoring is carried out, and where pain is treated with nitrates and narcotics, and anticoagulation therapy may be instituted. Hypertension and hypotension are treated appropriately. This has been a standard treatment for acute myocardial infarction for the last three decades. However, with the evolution of the heart catheterization laboratory into a therapeutic facility, the clinician is acutely aware of the opportunity to save life and salvage the myocardium by a more aggressive approach. The clinical circumstances determine how aggressive this approach should be.

The illustrations shown on the next page are from a 49 year old school teacher who presented with severe, unrelenting precordial pain. This was accompanied by hypotension. The ECG changes were characteristic of acute anterior wall transmural myocardial infarction. The patient was studied as an emergency and was found to have a large thrombus occluding the proximal left anterior descending coronary artery. Ten thousand units of intracoronary streptokinase was injected as a bolus and started drip at 2000 units per minute with reperfusion of the myocardium after half an hour of infusion and resolution of the acute changes. The shock relented as did the pain and the re-study of the coronaries showed a stenosis of about 60 to 70%. The patient enjoyed an uneventful recovery and was discharged on vasodilator therapy.

B. Intervention for Acute Coronary Occlusion

1. *Thrombolytic Therapy with Streptokinase*

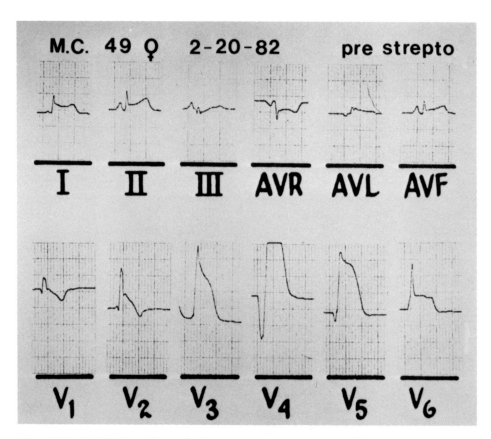

Fig. 111. A, ECG on day of admission showing ST-T elevation in the precordial leads, consistent with acute evolving anteroseptal infarction. Fig. 111 used with permission of The C. V. Mosby Company from Vlodaver Z., Boyum A., Gesundheit S., Long S., Peterson R., Spenny E., Thorsen R. D. Heart and Lung, 12:351, 1983.

B. Intervention for Acute Coronary Occlusion

1. *Thrombolytic Therapy with Streptokinase*

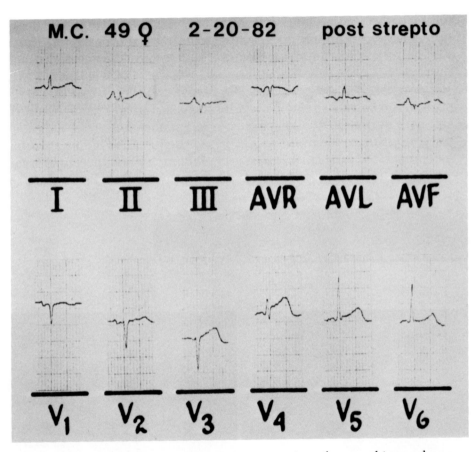

Fig. 111. B, ECG following intracoronary injection of streptokinase shows normalization of the ST-T segment elevation, but persistence of Q waves of the infarcted tissue.

C. Surgery for Impending Infarction

1. *Transluminal Balloon Angioplasty*

Shown on this and the next page are illustrations from a 61 year old male who began experiencing severe chest pain with mild exercise. This finally increased to a point where he was incapacitated by pain on slight exertion. The resting ECG was unremarkable. The patient was felt to represent a case of impending infarction. A coronary angiogram was performed on the fifth day of admission revealing a 95% stenosis of the right coronary artery. The other two coronary arteries were normal. The cardiac enzymes were normal. During the following morning the patient had two more episodes of angina at rest and he underwent transluminal balloon angioplasty with complete resolution of the obstruction and a return of the coronary artery to a normal calibre. The painful episodes subsided and the patient was discharged on the fourth hospital day.

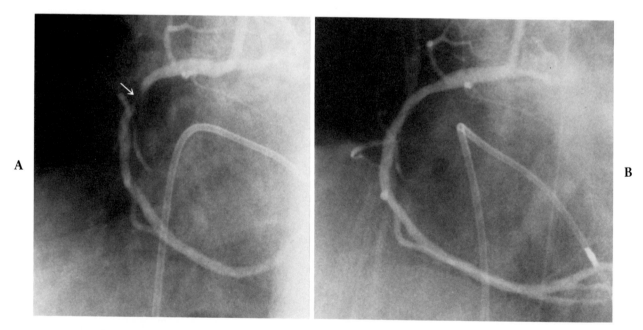

Fig. 114. A, RC arteriogram showing severe stenosis of the proximal segment (arrow). **B,** Following transluminal balloon angioplasty, the RC shows resolution of the obstruction and excellent reperfusion of the distal artery.

C. Surgery for Impending Infarction

2. *Intra-Aortic Balloon Pump*

A 60 year old white female was admitted to the hospital complaining of severe, frequent episodes of chest pain coming on at rest and only partially relieved by nitroglycerin. In addition she had a disturbance of her vision and had carotid bruits bilaterally. She had peripheral vascular disease. Because of the persistence of pain and fear of impending infarction, she had an intra-aortic balloon pump inserted on the sixth hospital day. She then underwent a carotid endarterectomy and triple saphenous vein graft bypass two weeks following admission.

Her postoperative course was characterized by slow recovery and poor healing of the leg wounds because of diffuse arteriosclerotic obstructive disease.

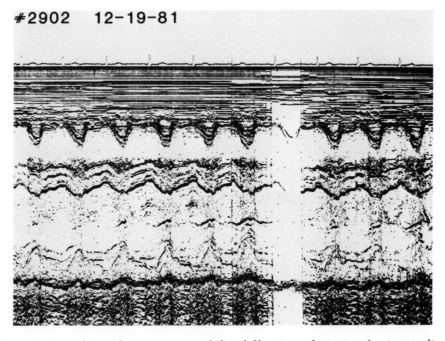

#2902   12-19-81

Fig. 115. LV echocardiogram, second day following admission for impending infarction, is unremarkable. Motion pattern of the IVS and PW within normal limits.

D. Surgery for Acutely Evolving Myocardial Infarction

When the patient has demonstrated an acute myocardial infarction by ECG and enzyme changes, the course of the disease may demand early investigation and possible surgical intervention. This situation was illustrated by a patient that sustained an acute anterior myocardial infarction and after two weeks was discharged from the hospital in stable condition. After only being home 24 hours, he was readmitted with recurrence of severe anterior chest pain. It was thought that the patient was either extending his original infarction or was having ischemic changes because of other coronary vessels that were significantly stenotic. The recurrent pain was initially relieved with analgesics but recurred the morning after admission. The pain became continuous and would not relent. An angiogram showed that the left main coronary had a 90% stenosis at its origin and there was a 50% stenosis in the distal left main coronary. The circumflex had a complete occlusion of the middle marginal branch. The posterior descending coronary was stenosed at the junction of the middle and distal third. The ventricular contractility was diminished. The inferior wall was very hypokinetic.

The patient was now in shock and an intra-aortic balloon pump was inserted with restoration of blood pressure to the level of 100 systolic with the use of inatropic agents as well. It was felt that the patient would not survive without surgical intervention. Both greater and lesser saphenous veins had been removed from both legs at prior operations. The internal mammary artery was taken down on both sides, the right being connected to the right coronary at the crux and the left being connected to the anterior descending at its midportion. The proximal left anterior descending and proximal left main were endarterectomized as was the branch leading to the septal perforator, the first diagonal and to the circumflex. It was possible to pass a probe into the aorta through the lumen of the left main after the endarterectomy. Blood pressure was low following bypass and this was in spite of the intra-aortic balloon.

D. Surgery for Acutely Evolving Myocardial Infarction

The patient fibrillated when the chest was closed and the chest was re-opened. Manual massage was carried out for about 20 minutes until bypass could be re-established. Then a left atrial to aortic assist device was used to unload the failing left ventricle. With this and the intra-aortic balloon and inatropic agents, the patient's chest could be closed and he was maintained for 16 hours. At the end of this time the myocardium no longer was contracting and the patient expired. Autopsy showed that there was an ostial stenosis of the left main coronary with somewhat of a flap valve obstructing the coronary orifice.

Comment: The mortality for patients in cardiogenic shock secondary to acute myocardial infarction is approximately 90%. Surgery, including emergency bypass with or without the help of the balloon pump and possible left ventricular assist devices, is capable of salvaging a small percentage of these patients. There have been a number of long term survivors, perhaps as high as 25% of patients who have been placed on left ventricular assist after being unable to maintain circulation with the balloon pump alone. The fatal outcome in this case of emergency surgery for extension of infarction and cardiogenic shock contrasts sharply with the similar clinical picture illustrated above where the acutely thrombosed left anterior descending coronary artery was opened with streptokinase and the ECG changes as well as the cardiogenic shock both relented.

D. Surgery for Acutely Evolving Myocardial Infarction

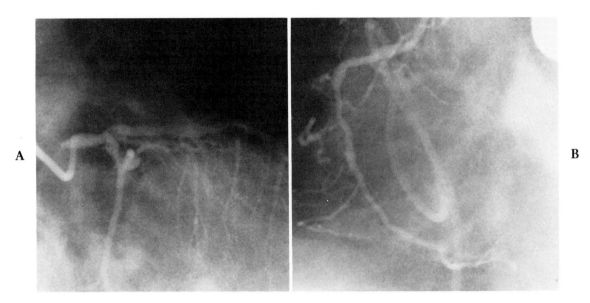

Fig. 116. A, LC arteriogram showing severe stenotic disease in the proximal segment of the LAD. **B,** RC arteriogram showing diffuse severe disease of the RC.

E. Surgery for Complications

1. *Ventricular Septal Rupture*

Ventricular septal rupture accompanies approximately 0.5 to 1.0% of all acute myocardial infarctions. This complication is suspected when the patient is convalescing from an acute myocardial infarction and develops a systolic murmur. The murmur must be distinguished from acute mitral insufficiency. The Swan-Ganz catheter in the right ventricle can be helpful in detecting a left-to-right shunt. Abnormally high oxygen concentrations in the right ventricle are characteristic of this left-to-right shunt. The patient may or may not tolerate the hemodynamic burden of the increased cardiac output associated with the defect.

A 58 year old developed epigastric pain and pain in both wrists. Four days later he returned to work and the epigastric pain and wrist pain returned again when he exerted himself. An acute myocardial infarction was diagnosed by enzyme and ECG changes and these indicated a transmural inferior myocardial infarction. He developed a loud systolic murmur heard best over the left precordium and it was suspected that he had either a ventricular septal defect, acquired, or mitral insufficiency. An urgent left ventriculogram was done showing a left-to-right shunt at the ventricular level with the shunt measured at 5 liters. The patient was digitalized and treated with diuretics and low salt diet and he was gradually able to ambulate. A repeat angiogram was done approximately six weeks from the time of the original myocardial infarction. This showed obstruction of the right coronary and inferior ventricular septal defect and evidence of left ventricular failure. This defect was closed with a patch. He convalesced uneventfully, returned to work for 10 years following surgery, when he developed exertional angina. An angiogram showed triple vessel coronary artery disease. There was persistence of the ventricular septal defect with a left-to-right shunt which was smaller than the original shunt and showed evidence of left ventricular failure. Surgery was not recommended because of the impairment of the left ventricle and the patient was treated medically for a time and finally sustained another myocardial infarction and died.

E. Surgery for Complications

1. *Ventricular Septal Rupture*

Comment: This individual developed a ventricular septal defect a few days after the onset of an acute myocardial infarction. He was managed medically for 10 weeks following his infarct and then the defect was closed but there was a residual that persisted for 10 years. He eventually developed additional symptoms of coronary insufficiency and, because of poor left ventricular function, he was not considered a surgical candidate.

E. Surgery for Complications

2. *Left Ventricular Aneurysm*

Left ventricular aneurysm complicates acute myocardial infarction in 5 to 15% of cases. The aneurysm may be either anterior or inferior in its location. It may be complicated by ventricular septal defect or it may occur in an isolated fashion. The aneurysm is significant because of three features. First, it may be associated with a thrombus which could embolize. It may be associated with such a mechanical disadvantage of decompressing the ventricle each time it contracts, that failure may result. It may also rupture. However, the last possibility is the least likely to occur. The following illustrates the clinical features of a very large left ventricular aneurysm.

A 68 year old white male retiree experienced severe anterior chest pain. He was hospitalized and had a cardiac arrest and was resuscitated. Five days later, he developed pulmonary edema, corrected with diuretics. At three weeks he was discharged to his home but became nauseated. He again developed pulmonary edema and was readmitted to the intensive care unit. After a few days at home he was admitted to another hospital where arteriography showed complete obstruction of the left anterior descending coronary artery with a large ballooning out of the left ventricle compatible with aneurysm. The right coronary artery was highly stenotic at its midportion. The circumflex looked normal. The patient was in borderline failure and an intra-aortic balloon pump was kept available but not used. At the time of surgery there was a hugely dilated left ventricle with aneurysm adherent to the surface of the pericardium. The pulmonary pressure was elevated. The aneurysm was filled with a clot which occupied the anterior one half of the left ventricle. The anterior and posterior papillary muscles were intact. The muscle of the anterior one half of the left ventricle was severely thinned out and lined with a heavy clot. The clot extended almost up to the aortic valve. The septum was intact. The aneurysm was resected and the edges of the cut ventricle were approximated with the use of Ivalon sponge buttressing mattress sutures. Saphenous vein graft was sewn to the right coronary beyond the obstruction. Following surgery, the patient was physically active and denied any symptoms. He remained on lanoxin, dyazide and aspirin. Eleven years later he continues to do well.

E. Surgery for Complications

2. *Left Ventricular Aneurysm*

Comment: This patient had cardiac cachexia with wasting of his extremities and was symptomatic at bed rest. The correction of the aneurysm permitted the ventricle to contract adequately and the patient resumed his normal life style.

E. Surgery for Complications

2. *Left Ventricular Aneurysm*

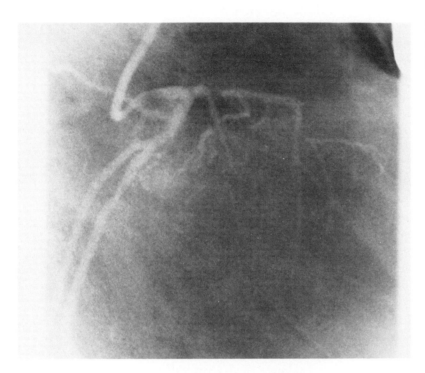

Fig. 117. LC arteriogram showing almost complete occlusion of the proximal LAD.

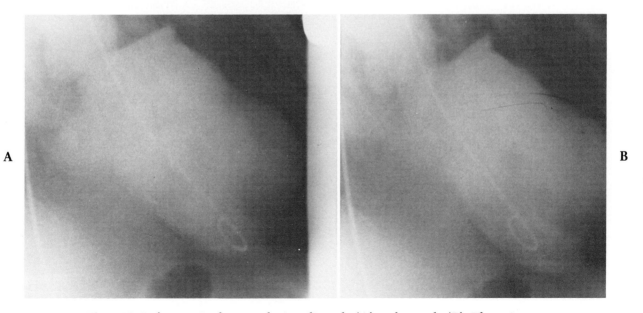

A   B

Fig. 118. Left ventriculogram during diastole (**A**) and systole (**B**). There is a distorted enlargement of an akinetic apical portion of the LV, the characteristic appearance of an LV aneurysm.

E. Surgery for Complications

3. *Acute Papillary Muscle Dysfunction*

A 53 year old white male office manager was admitted to the hospital with an acute myocardial infarction. He was well until the day of admission. He had low back and flank pain as well as nausea, sweating and diaphoresis. The paramedics noted that the patient was in atrial fibrillation with the rate of 40 to 60. The fibrillation dropped to 30 to 40 beats per minute when admitted to the emergency room. This was treated with atropine and also the ventricular irritability was treated with lidocaine. Auscultation revealed apical S-4 and no murmur. The CPK was 4,560 and LDH 652. Atrial flutter developed on the fifth day after admission. This lead to atrial fibrillation with rapid ventricular response. Atrial flutter persisted at the rate of 140 to 160 and hypotension developed. Emergency cardioversion was performed and sinus tachycardia resulted. Over the next six hours left ventricular failure developed with basilar rates and increased pulmonary congestion on the chest x-ray. He also developed a high pitched mid-apical systolic murmur with no associated heave or lift. It was felt that the patient had mitral regurgitation secondary to papillary muscle dysfunction or rupture of the chordae. Diuretics produced diuresis, atrial flutter and fibrillation recurred and cardioversion was again attempted without success. A Swan-Ganz catheter revealed pulmonary artery pressure of 43/20 with a wedge of 23 and prominent V wave on the tracing. The echocardiogram showed left ventricular enlargement with failure, borderline left atrial enlargement, systolic prolapse of the mitral valve with no flail leaflets. An intra-aortic balloon was inserted. A heart catheterization was performed and there was no evidence of left-to-right shunt. The left ventriculogram showed severe mitral regurgitation. The basal half of the inferior wall was non-contractile. The degree of mitral regurgitation was sufficient to fill the atrial appendage and pulmonary veins. The remainder of the ventricle contracted well. There was total occlusion of the right coronary near its origin. The left diagonal coronary artery was 75% narrowed. The anterior descending, circumflex left main coronary arteries were normal. The left ventricular end diastolic pressure was 18.

E. Surgery for Complications

3. *Acute Papillary Muscle Dysfunction*

The patient was operated on the day of the heart catheterization. He had an episode of ventricular tachycardia at the induction of anesthesia that responded to one direct current shock. The inferior wall of the left ventricle did not contract. The mitral valve papillary muscles were thinned out, pale and the chordae were stretched. The posterior leaflet appeared unusually fragile. The anterior leaflet looked fairly normal. The valve was replaced with a #27 Bjork-Shiley tilting disk prosthesis and the left diagonal and right coronary arteries were bypassed. The patient had atrial tachyarrhythmias complicating his otherwise smooth postoperative course and he remained on lanoxin and diuretics as well as anticoagulants at the time of discharge. Three years later he remains free of symptoms and is carrying out his normal activities.

E. Surgery for Complications

3. *Acute Papillary Muscle Dysfunction*

Comments: This patient sustained an inferior myocardial infarction. Early in the post infarction state he developed evidence of left ventricular dysfunction and a Swan-Ganz catheter clearly indicated this to be a mitral insufficiency rather than a ventricular septal defect. A balloon pump was required to stabilize the patient before angiography and during induction for mitral valve replacement and coronary artery bypass.

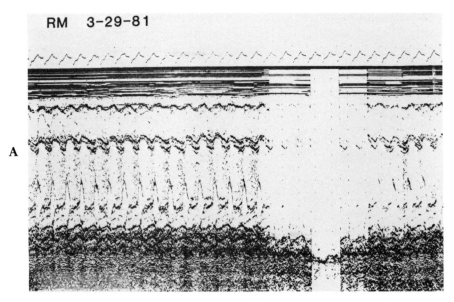

Fig. 119. A, LV echocardiogram before surgery, shows enlarged LV, mild enlarged LA, hypokinesis and thinning of the PW and small prolapse of the mitral valve. LVD: 73mm. LA: 45 mm. EF: 44%

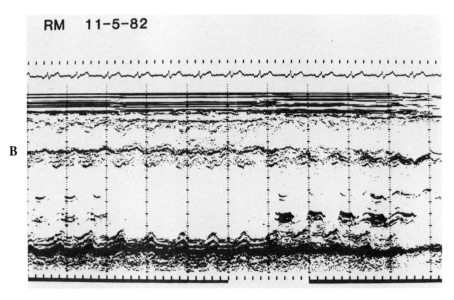

Fig. 119. B, Twenty months following surgery the LV echocardiogram shows LV and LA smaller, mitral valve replaced by a prosthetic valve (#27 Bjork-Shiley tilting disk valve) and LV function improved. LVD: 62 mm. LA: 38 mm. EFL 55%

E. Surgery for Complications

3. *Acute Papillary Muscle Dysfunction*

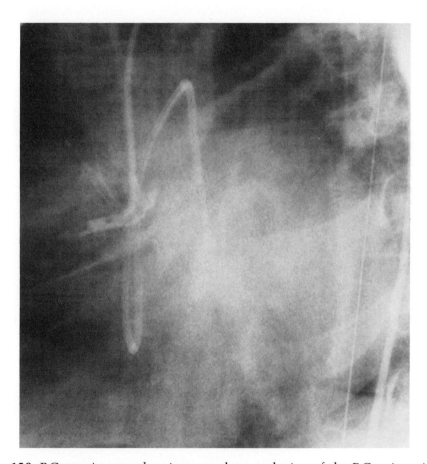

Fig. 120. RC arteriogram showing complete occlusion of the RC at its origin.

E. Surgery for Complications

4. *Cardiogenic Shock*

Approximately 15% of patients sustaining acute myocardial infarction developed cardiogenic shock. This is defined as systolic pressure less than 90 mm of mercury, a urine output of less than 25 cc per hour. The patient is best managed by insertion of a Swan-Ganz catheter to measure the filling pressure of the left ventricle. Sometimes there is a lack of adequate filling, possibly related to the use of diuretics and this can be judiciously corrected by the infusion of crystaloid or colloid solutions. The central venous pressure by itself is not as accurate as the wedge pressure of the Swan-Ganz catheter in determining whether or not the adequate filling volumes are present. If these volumes are adequate and the patient remains in shock, the use of inatropic agents such as dopamine or dobutrex is helpful. If these fail to maintain adequate pressure, then the use of an intra-aortic balloon would be the next modality to support the failing cardiac output. The balloon pump reduces the pressure against which the left ventricle must open to eject its contents and thus reduces somewhat the work of the heart. It also increases the pressure of perfusion after the aortic valve closes, thus increasing the coronary perfusion pressure and coronary volume. The balloon pump supports the circulation and gives the cardiologist time to study the coronary anatomy. If correctable lesions are discovered, then either balloon dilatation or streptokinase or coronary bypass surgery is indicated. The patient is seldom able to be sufficiently benefitted by balloon pumping alone as a definitive form of treatment.

E. Surgery for Complications

4. *Cardiogenic Shock*

A 65 year old white male, retired business executive developed progressively severe anterior chest pain starting 10 days before admission. The pains were relieved by nitroglycerin sublingually but pain would recur quickly. He was hospitalized and an acute myocardial infarction was ruled out. Because of recurrence of pain he was returned to the coronary care unit. He experienced sudden and unexpected ventricular fibrillation. He was immediately resuscitated. He remained cold and clammy but alert and cooperative. Blood pressure was between 60 and 80 systolic but could be elevated to 90 with aramine. The electrocardiogram showed no change in the pattern of acute myocardial infarction. An intra-aortic balloon was inserted and with it the pressure was able to be maintained at 80 to 90 mm of mercury. A coronary anteriogram showed 70% stenosis of the left anterior descending proximal to the diagonal and with virtually total occlusion distal to the diagonal. There was delayed opacification of the distal three quarters of the left anterior descending. There was retrograde filling of the right posterior descending via the left marginal and left diagonal branches. The opacification of the right coronary showed complete occlusion near its origin. The left ventriculogram showed a large dyskinetic area involving the distal two thirds of the anterior wall and apex and distal third of the inferior wall. There was marked increase in the residual volume with reduced ejection fraction. The left ventricular end diastolic pressure was elevated at rest and rose to 28 mm of mercury after the ventriculogram. The patient was operated on as an emergency. The anterior surface of the left ventricle did not contract. The tip of the left ventricle was very fragile and softened, measuring 2 cm in diameter near the tip. There was old scarring of the diaphragmatic surface of the left ventricle. The infarcted area of the left ventricle was imbricated. The left anterior descending and the right coronary arteries were bypassed using saphenous vein grafts. The patient enjoyed a relatively smooth postoperative course except that a partial disruption of the sternum developed which was repaired a year after surgery. Subsequently the patient has enjoyed a fairly normal life.

E. Surgery for Complications

4. *Cardiogenic Shock*

Comment: This case illustrates the development of cardiogenic shock approximately 10 days after the onset of an acute anterior myocardial infarction. The infarcted area was fairly circumscribed. It was possible to revascularize both the left anterior descending coronary and right coronary. This contributed to his prompt recovery from cardiogenic shock.

E. Surgery for Complications

4. *Cardiogenic Shock*

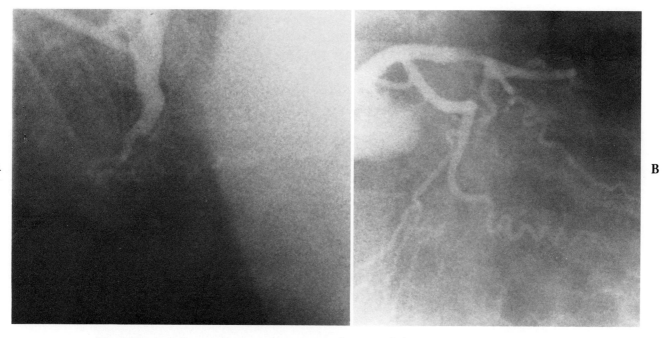

Fig. 121. A, RC arteriogram showing occlusion of the RC near its origin.
B, LC arteriogram shows severe stenosis of the LAD proximal to the diagonal
branch and total occlusion distal to that branch.

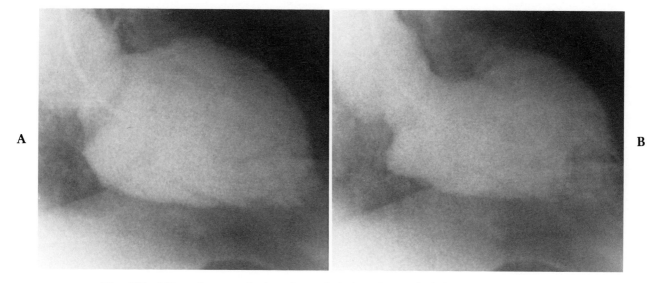

Fig. 122. LV angiogram during diastole (**A**) and systole (**B**), demonstrating
akinesis of the anteroapical segment of the LV and distal third of the inferior
wall.

F. Echocardiographic Evaluation After Coronary Bypass Surgery

The use of M-mode and two-dimensional echocardiography in patients after coronary bypass surgery is a reliable method for identifying areas of abnormal motion and contraction of segments in the LV wall, and for assessing their reversibility. About 6 to 10% of the patients after coronary bypass surgery may develop new Q waves in the electrocardiograms, and the echocardiograms in these cases may show dyskinesis of the IV septum or inferior wall in the M-mode study, with relatively normal or mildly reduced LV function values.

The LV echocardiographic patterns normalize in most of these patients within three months after surgery.

ECG changes of new Q waves that follow coronary bypass surgery are possibly the result of focal areas of injury, often microscopic, and multifocal, that heal and normalize completely three months after surgery.

With two-dimensional echocardiography study, abnormal segmental motion and thinned echo-dense infarcted areas of scar tissue, are unlikely to have their function restored.

But areas with motion abnormalities, and normal diastolic thickness, may restore their function after coronary bypass surgery.

F. Echocardiographic Evaluation After Coronary Bypass Surgery

Shown on this page are illustrations from a patient with a history of subendocardial lateral infarction, and recent coronary bypass surgery, with significant improvement in exercise tolerance and LV function following a long term exercise conditioning program.

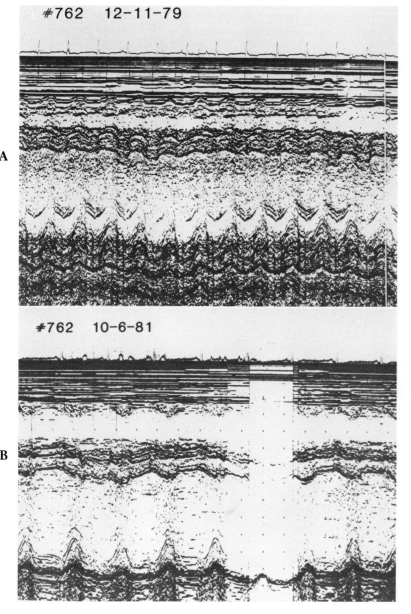

Fig. 123. A, M-mode LV echocardiogram two weeks following surgery, showing dyskinesis of the IVS. EF: 62%; level of exercise activity: 3 METS.

Fig. 123. B, One and a half years after surgery, the M-mode LV study shows improvement in motion and systolic thickening of the IVS. LVD: 53mm; EF: 71%; level of exercise activity: 7½ METS.

F. Echocardiographic Evaluation After Coronary Bypass Surgery

Illustrations from a patient with subendocardial inferior wall infarction and recent coronary bypass surgery, with improved motion and contraction pattern of the inferior wall after the procedure.

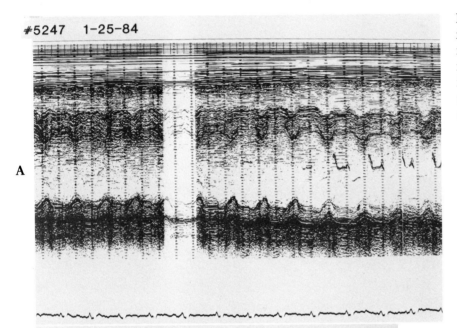

Fig. 124. A, LV echocardiogram four days after admission for acute myocardial infarction. Shows reduced systolic thickening of the inferior wall. Normal motion of the IVS. EF: 61%; thickening of the PW: 30%.

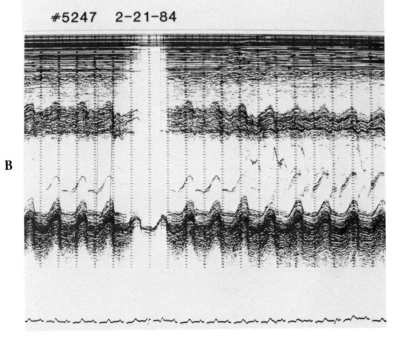

Fig. 124. B, Three weeks after coronary bypass surgery, motion of the inferior wall and systolic thickening improved. Paradoxic motion of the IVS, new since previous study prior to surgery. EF: 65%; thickening of the PW: 45%.

F. Echocardiographic Evaluation After Coronary Bypass Surgery

Illustrations from a patient with history of angina and recent coronary bypass surgery. New small Q waves developed in the ECG in leads V1 through V3.

Following surgery, patient was asymptomatic during exercise activities, exercise tolerance improved, and LV echocardiographic pattern normalized three months later. Patient participated in an outpatient cardiac exercise program.

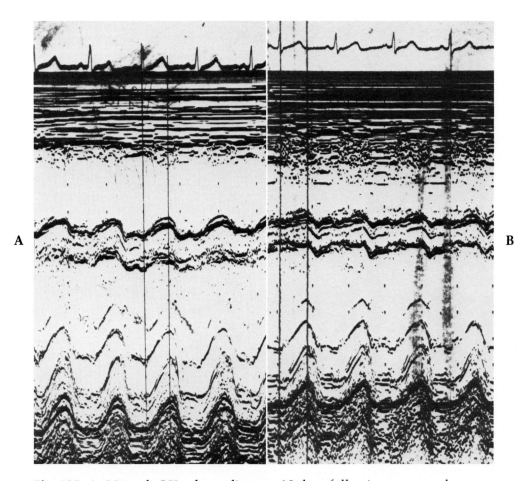

Fig. 125. A, M-mode LV echocardiogram 10 days following coronary bypass surgery, showing paradoxical motion of the IVS. LVD: 45mm; EF: 57%; level of exercise activity: 3 METS. **B,** Three months after participating in a cardiac outpatient exercise program. The LV echocardiogram shows improvement in motion pattern of the IVS. LVD: 48mm; EF: 61%; level of exercise activity: 5 METS.

F. Echocardiographic Evaluation After Coronary Bypass Surgery

Shown on this and the next page are illustrations from a patient with previous extensive anteroseptal infarction, and recent coronary bypass surgery. Three months following the surgical procedure, patient exercise tolerance and LV function improved significantly. The size of the LV is smaller, the motion of the IV septum less dyskinetic.

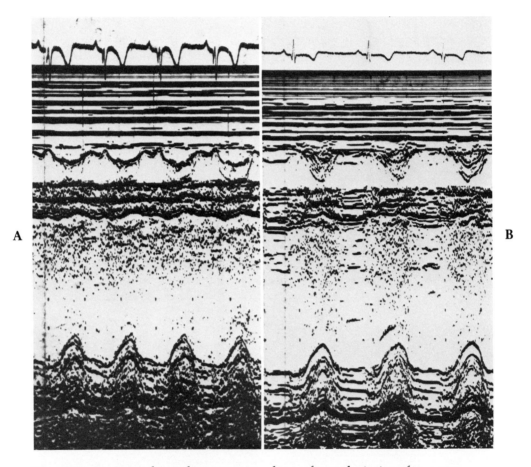

Fig. 126. A, LV echocardiogram two days after admission for acute anteroseptal infarction, showing hypokinesis and reduced systolic thickening of the IV septum. LVD: 56mm; EF: 33%; level of exercise activity: 1½ METS. **B,** LV echocardiogram three months later, showing some improvement in LV function, the IV septum remains hypokinetic, and there is reduced systolic thickening. LVD: 56mm; EF: 55%; level of exercise activity: 3 METS. ECG monitoring showed ST-T segment depression during exercise activity, associated with chest pain.

F. Echocardiographic Evaluation After Coronary Bypass Surgery

Illustrations from the patient shown on previous page, following coronary bypass surgery for coronary insufficiency post myocardial infarction.

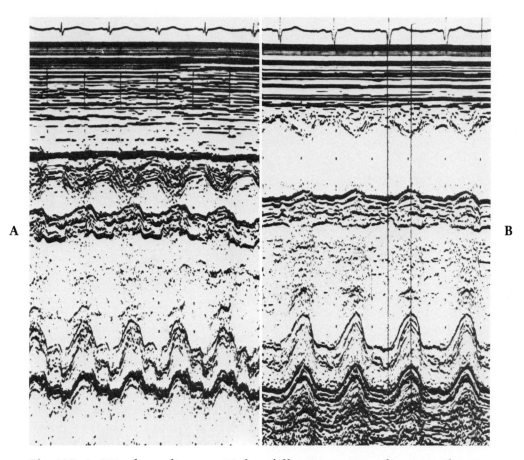

Fig. 127. A, LV echocardiogram, 10 days following surgery, showing reduction in the size of the LV, and paradoxical motion of the IVS. LVD: 44mm; EF: 55%; level of exercise activity: 3 METS. **B,** Three months later, the IVS is less dyskinetic; LV function is improved. LVD: 45mm; EF: 68%; level of exercise activity: 5½ METS. Patient asymptomatic during exercise; ST-T segment and ECG monitoring were stable.

F. Echocardiographic Evaluation After Coronary Bypass Surgery

Illustrations from a patient with previous extensive inferoseptal infarction, and recent coronary bypass surgery, with improved LV function and exercise tolerance, and the echocardiographic motion pattern unchanged.

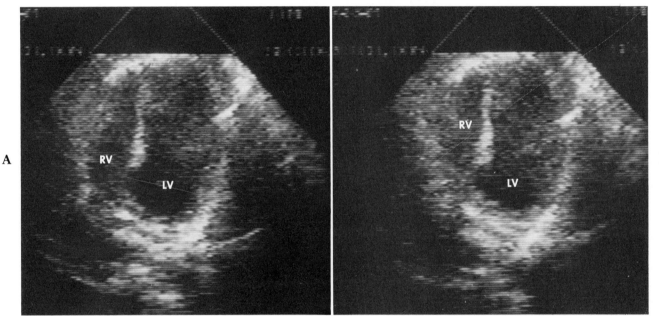

Fig. 128. A, Seven days after admission for acute inferior wall infarction. Two-dimensional echocardiogram, apical four-chamber view with inferior angulation, shows thinning and some dilatation of the inferoseptal segment of the LV. EF: 56%. **B,** Apical four-chamber view, 14 days following coronary bypass surgery, the area of thinning and dilation of the inferoseptal segment of the LV is unchanged. EF: 62%. Patient is asymptomatic and has improved exercise tolerance.

F. Echocardiographic Evaluation After Coronary Bypass Surgery

Shown on this page are illustrations from a patient with a history of previous infarction, and a recent acute infarction complicating coronary bypass surgery. His exercise tolerance was reduced, and LV function impaired, following the procedure.

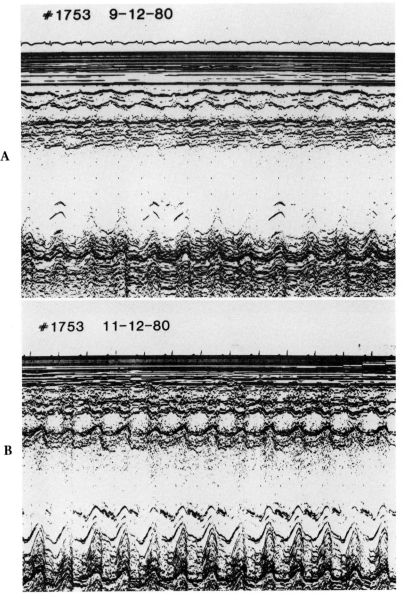

Fig. 129. A, LV echocardiogram, two days after admission for acute anteroseptal infarction, showing akinesis of the IVS. LVD: 63%; ejection time: 0.280 sec; LV EF: 40%; mean VCF: 0.57 cm/sec; thickening of the septum: 0; thickening of the PW: 30%; level of exercise activity: 1½ METS.

Fig. 129. B, LV echocardiogram, 10 days following coronary bypass surgery complicated with acute infarction. There is paradoxic motion of the IVS, the size of the LV is enlarged, and relatively hyperkinetic PW. EF: 46%.

F. Echocardiographic Evaluation After Coronary Bypass Surgery

The development of pericardial thickening changes, and small effusion related to the surgical procedure, are very common following coronary bypass surgery. Usually these pericardial changes are minimal, with non-significant hemodynamic implications. Shown on this page is a rare case of severe pericardial effusion developed after coronary bypass surgery, with clinical signs of constriction, making necessary pericardiocentesis to drain the accumulation of the effusion. Following this procedure, patient's exercise tolerance improve significantly.

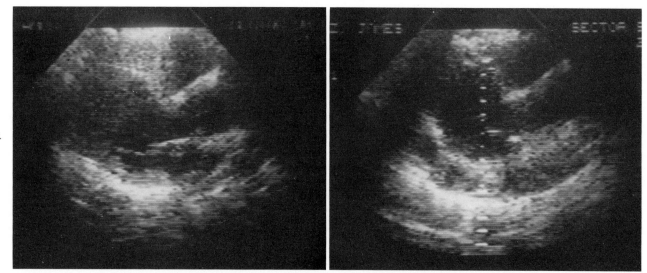

A   **B**

Fig. 130. **A**, Parasternal long axis view. Two-dimensional echocardiogram one week following admission for coronary insufficiency. Size of the chambers, and pericardium within normal. In real time, there was mild hypokinesis of the IV septum. **B**, Parasternal long axis view, 10 days following coronary bypass surgery showing small effusion in the pericardium.

F. Echocardiographic Evaluation After Coronary Bypass Surgery

Illustrations from the patient shown on previous page, with large effusion developing after coronary bypass surgery.

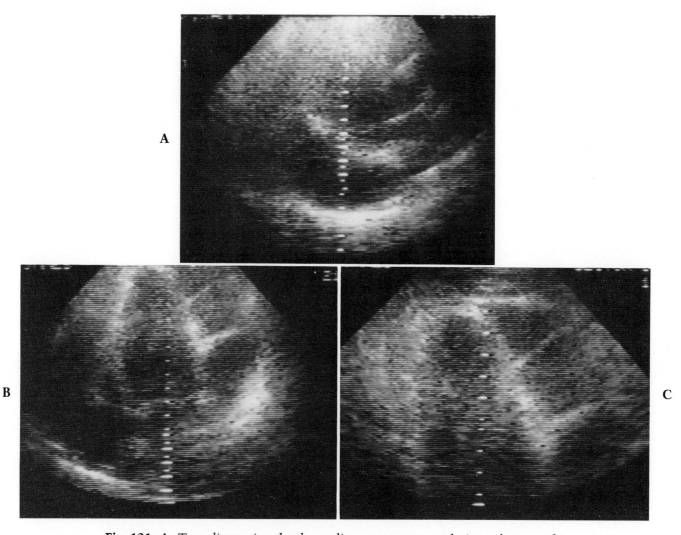

Fig. 131. **A,** Two-dimensional echocardiogram, parasternal view, three weeks following coronary bypass surgery, showing increased and large effusion in the pericardium. **B,** Apical four-chamber view, showing large effusion and fibrinous bands in the pericardial sac, representing organizational changes in the effusion. **C,** Close up view of the fibrinous bands in the pericardial fluid.

MODIFICATION OF RISK FACTORS

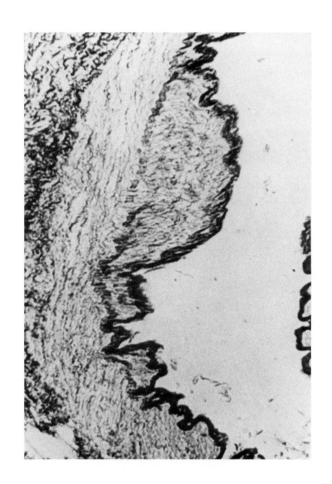

It is generally accepted that atherosclerosis begins in childhood and progresses in adolescence and young adulthood, even though serious clinical manifestation does not appear until middle age or later.

At the time of birth, the coronary arteries have not attained their maximal development. The intima and elastic tissue grow progressively from birth to old age.

In fetuses the intima is a thin layer lying upon an internal elastic membrane which is an uninterrupted distinct sheath.

Alterations of the fetal characteristics, which begin a few days after birth, consist of localized splitting and fragmentation of the internal elastic membrane and proliferation of fibroblasts.

During the first postnatal month, progressive longitudinal splitting of the internal elastic membrane occurs and, in the spaces between the splits, smooth muscle-like cells begin to appear, and a new layer between the media and intima, the so-called musculo-elastic layer, forms focally.

In cross-sections, focal protrusions into the lumen may be observed, representing the newly formed musculo-elastic layer with its overlying thickened intima.

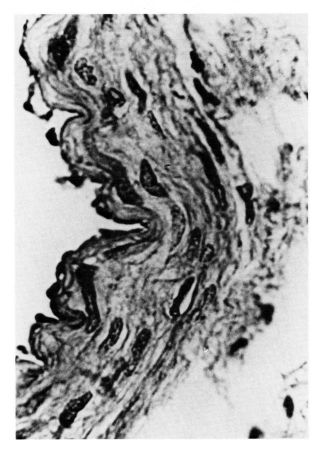

Fig. 132. Coronary artery from a premature stillborn female infant. The intima consists of a very thin layer of endothelial cells, the internal elastic membrane is intact, the media consists of delicate smooth muscle cells with occasional delicate elastic fibrils. Hematoxylin and eosin × 165. (From Vlodaver et al. *Academic Press*, 1975). Fig. 132 used with permission of Academic Press, Inc. from Coronary Arterial Variations in the Normal Heart and in Congenital Heart Disease, New York, 1975. by Vlodaver Z., Neufeld H. N., and Edwards J. E.

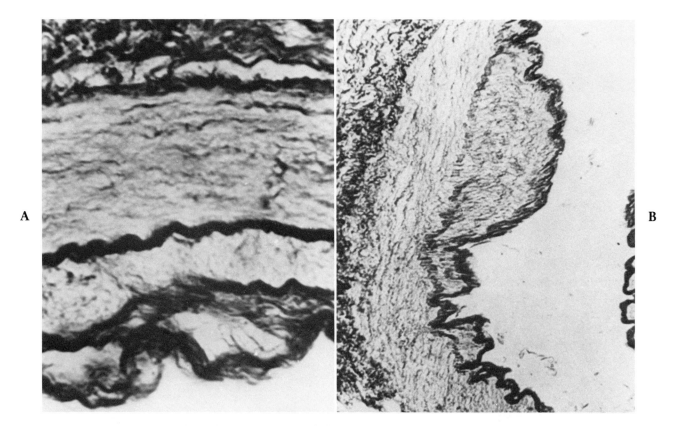

Fig. 133. A, Histologic structure of the coronary arteries in infants. Splitting of the internal elastic membrane, from an infant, two months old. Elastic tissue stain ×235. **B,** Cushion-like structures formed by proliferation of fibroelastic tissue, from a three day old infant. Elastic tissue stain ×56.

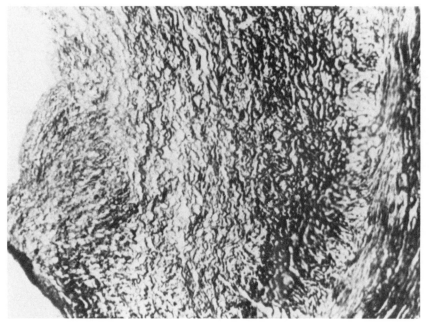

Fig. 134. Localized thickening of the intima, in the coronary artery from a seven year old boy. Elastic tissue stain ×146.
Fig. 134 used with permission of Academic Press Inc, from Coronary Arterial Variations in the Normal Heart and in Congenital Heart Disease, New York, 1975 by Vlodaver Z., Neufeld H.N., and Edwards J.E.

These morphologic alterations apparently result from many endogenous (sex or inheritance) and exogenous factors.

It is assumed that the most important factors affecting the structure are mechanical and/or metabolic in infants and children as a whole, as well as localized in the tissues of the coronary arterial wall itself.

Some investigators believe that the earliest demonstrable alterations, the splitting of the internal elastic membrane and associated focal proliferation of cells, represent reactions of the vessel to the hemodynamic stresses of the early postnatal state.

Others believe that the intimal thickening in the early ages is not to be interpreted as a natural developmental phenomenon, but rather as an abnormal process and a forerunner of the atherosclerotic process, and call the early intimal changes "pre-atheroma".

Differences in the intensity and quantity of the structural findings between the sexes and among various ethnic groups are found in early life.

Statistical analysis shows the intimal thickening of the coronary arteries in early life to be more developed in the Ashkenazy male than in the Yemenite and Bedouin males. This correlates closely with the prevalence of coronary heart disease in the corresponding adult population in these three ethnic groups.

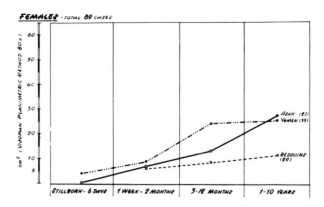

Fig. 135. Mean values of measurements of intima and musculo-elastic layer in coronary arteries of female children in three ethnic groups. No significant differences were founded. Fig. 135 used with permission of the American Heart Association Inc. From Vlodaver Z., Kahn H. A., and Neufeld H. N. Circulation 39:541, 1969.

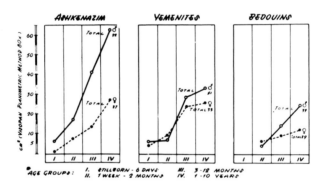

Fig. 136. Mean values of measurements of intima and musculoelastic layer in coronary arteries in three ethnic groups. Comparison between males and females in 211 cases, shows thickening of the coronary arteries in early life to be more pronounced among Ashkenazy male than in the Yemenite and Bedouin male. This was not true for females. These differences are apparent soon after birth, but are more obvious at the end of the first year of life.

The intimal tissue in the Ashkenazy males is more developed than in Ashkenazy females. This was not true for the other ethnic groups.
Fig. 136 used with permission of the American Heart Association Inc. From Vlodaver Z., Kahn H. A., and Neufeld H. N. Circulation 39:541, 1969.

INDEX